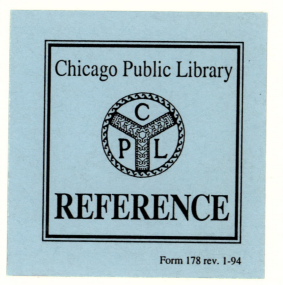

the

Perimenopause handbook

*What Every Woman
Needs to Know About the
Years Before Menopause*

Carol Turkington

CB

CONTEMPORARY BOOKS

Library of Congress Cataloging-in-Publication Data

Turkington, Carol.
  The perimenopause handbook: what every woman needs to
know about the years before menopause / Carol Turkington ;
foreword by Susan Johnson.
      p.   cm.
  Includes bibliographical references.
  ISBN 0-8092-2935-8
  1. Perimenopause—Popular works.   I. Title.
RG188.T87   1998
618.1'75—dc21   97-51584
                                                            CIP

Cover design by Monica Baziuk
Interior design by PageMasters & Company

Published by Contemporary Books
A division of NTC/Contemporary Publishing Group, Inc.
4255 West Touhy Avenue, Lincolnwood (Chicago), Illinois 60646-1975 U.S.A.
Printed in the United States of America
International Standard Book Number: 0-8092-2935-8
98   99   00   01   02   03   QP   6   5   4   3   2   1

꧁꧂

For Wanda Miller

Also by Carol Turkington

Contents

Foreword

"Perimenopause" has always been a nebulous term in the medical lexicon. In fact, after almost two decades as a gynecologist, with the most recent years spent specializing in menopause, even I could never quite tell what the authors of medical articles meant by the term! In a literal sense, menopause means the last menstrual period—and I think most women would agree that this single event, while important, is not nearly the whole story.

*Peri*menopause, on the other hand, refers to the time around menopause—a much more interesting and useful concept, since women have always known that lots of things happen for several years before and after this event. However, until very recently no one had thought to study what really went on during that time, and so health care providers could offer little helpful advice or information to women experiencing perimenopause. Coupled with the fact that many women were reluctant to discuss their physiological changes, women entering this phase have been at a real disadvantage.

Fortunately, things have begun to change. This is in part due to increased public openness about the subject, and also in part due to the pioneering efforts of a few groups of medical investigators. Readers will perhaps not be surprised to learn that these groups have typically been led by women scientists. These studies have provided important new information and raised intriguing new questions as well.

Carol Turkington makes this newfound information accessible to all women, and she clearly presents the numerous options available for women who need advice about troublesome symptoms. This is a wonderful service, particularly since in my experience many health care providers have not yet been educated in this area. Perimenopause is a normal part of life. Armed with accurate information, and with access to appropriate health care options if necessary, women can approach this time of their life with confidence.

—Susan R. Johnson, M.D., M.S.
Associate Dean for Faculty Affairs & Professor of Obstetrics and Gynecology, University of Iowa, College of Medicine

Acknowledgments

The creation of any book always involves a wide variety of people, and this one is no exception. I'd like to thank staffers at the National Library of Medicine and the medical libraries of the Hershey Medical Center, the University of Pennsylvania Medical Center, and the National Institutes of Health.

I also appreciate the personal input and advice from a wide number of women, including Susan Johnson, M.D., M.S., Wanda Miller, Sarah Fisher, and the moms at Lancaster Country Day School.

Finally, I'd like to thank Susan Schwartz at NTC/Contemporary Publishing for her expert editorial guidance, Bert Holtje of James Peter Associates for valuable support, and, as always, Michael and Kara.

Introduction

Within the next ten years, 21 million American women of the baby boom generation will enter perimenopause—that's almost 6,000 women a day. In boardrooms and living rooms across the country, we represent the largest group of American women in history to enter this reproductive phase all at once. Yet this time of life remains a mystery to many women.

Many of us will be confused, surprised, and disturbed as we begin to experience memory problems, poor concentration, hot flashes, headaches, moodiness, and weight gain. Too many of us have little idea about what is going on inside our bodies. Until very recently perimenopause was just not something that doctors took very seriously or that scientists bothered to study, and so we may be unprepared for the chronic, prolonged symptoms of the premenopausal period.

For menopause is not a sudden event. We don't go to bed one night with fully functional ovaries and then wake up the next morning in menopause. Instead, menopause is a process of gradual change that begins many years before the fifth decade of life.

This early stage of menopause, called "perimenopause," often begins during a woman's 30s as the ovaries slow down and estrogen levels drop. By the mid-40s women may notice signs of estrogen withdrawal (mood swings or hot flashes). But because many women think of menopause as the time when they stop having periods, those in perimenopause—who are still having their periods—don't connect these early symptoms with menopause at all. The irritability or memory problems are often ascribed to tension, stress, a bad day, or PMS.

If we get as far as our doctor's office with these complaints, all too often we may be told that because we're still menstruating, we are "too young" to be in menopause. Many doctors today still believe that as long as a woman has periods, her complaints must have nothing to do with menopause. Too many doctors are still willing to shrug off many of the perimenopausal symptoms as something that is "all in a woman's head."

When Sherry, 43, asked her doctor if her moodiness and "brain fog" were related to early menopause, she was told that because she was still having her period, she couldn't be having menopausal symptoms. The fact that she was irritable, moody, and was experiencing vaginal dryness and memory problems didn't add up to "menopause" to these health care workers. Sherry wanted a hormone test because she wanted to get an early start on managing her perimenopausal symptoms, but she was told "We won't check your hormone levels unless you've stopped having your periods or you're having hot flashes. You're too young to be menopausal."

Fortunately, researchers are beginning to realize that to better understand menopause, they do need to start looking at women in their 30s and 40s, the time when the most noticeable symptoms of menopause begin. Unlike earlier generations, more and more women are speaking up about their symptoms and demanding answers about what they can do to prepare for the change.

For those of us who go through the process early, it's vital to understand what's happening to our bodies *now*, when we still have time to make good choices that can affect our health in the future. By the time more severe symptoms appear, changes have already been going on for months—or even years.

There is a wide range of health problems related to the onset of menopause, including osteoporosis, heart disease, and breast cancer. There are ways to minimize those risks—but first we must realize they exist. It's important to discuss the health choices and decisions we can make today that may significantly impact our health for months and years in the future. Eating a good diet, taking vitamin supplements, learning to relax, exercising, quitting smoking, and not drinking too much—all these lifestyle decisions can have a real impact on how healthy we'll be in the next 20 or 30 years.

It's not what we do by the time we're menopausal, but what we do to prepare for it that can make the difference between good health and crippling disability.

1 What Is Perimenopause?

Karen was a 42-year-old financial planner who was not especially concerned when her periods became irregular. But then she noticed that throughout the day she was experiencing rushes of heat that left her uncomfortable and sweating. She began to have problems with sleeping. She seemed to be spending all her time in the bathroom, and she struggled to remember the names of her clients. This "brain fog" was the scariest symptom of all. Her mother had died just two years before of Alzheimer's disease. Was Karen going to end up like her mother, frightened and confused?

Her symptoms seemed like menopause—but she was much too young to be going through the change, she thought. "I was afraid I was losing my mind, or that I was starting to get Alzheimer's too," she recalls.

Her next period flow was so heavy, Karen feared she was hemorrhaging. Her gynecologist reassured her: She wasn't bleeding abnormally, and she didn't have Alzheimer's. She was experiencing something called "perimenopause."

More and more experts are starting to pay attention to the perimenopause—those years leading up to menopause that can begin as early as the mid-30s, or as late as the early 50s. Menopause itself is defined as when a woman stops menstruating for at least 12 months.

We're hearing more about this introduction to menopause because experts have begun to realize that menopause isn't so much an abrupt health event as it is a gradual process of aging that occurs when your body begins to shift gears as the reproductive years pass. Symptoms can appear up to 15 years before menopause begins; other women go through the early stages of perimenopause in just a month.

Some lucky women—about 20 percent—have such an easy time of it they don't notice perimenopause at all and are completely unaware of the gradual decrease in hormones as their body begins to gear down. Another 5 to 10 percent have minor problems (maybe a few irregular periods or a couple of hot flashes). But 10 to 35 percent of women experience severe, long-lasting symptoms, including irregular periods, hot flashes, insomnia, mood swings, and breast tenderness. For these women the symptoms are much like having a constant bout of premenstrual syndrome (PMS), and can seriously interfere with their daily lives.

The problem is that because many women think of menopause as the month their periods finally stop, they don't often connect these symptoms with hormonal changes. Women may believe they are suffering from PMS, from stress-related irritability, or from age-related memory loss. Just as they begin to see their vision worsen because of age-related eye changes, they assume that short-term memory loss must mean the beginning of Alzheimer's disease.

Those women who become concerned enough to see their doctor may still be told that "you're too young to be in menopause," reflecting the common notion that either you're menopausal or you're not. If you're still having periods, some physicians still will tell you that your symptoms must be either due to another cause, or "all in your head."

What Happens in Your Body

Starting in your preteen or teenage years, each month your body releases one of the more than 400,000 eggs stored in your ovaries—as well as the layer of cells that cover the egg. The covering layer of cells surrounding these eggs is the primary producer of the hormones estrogen and progesterone.

These primary hormones involved in the beginning of menstruation are follicle-stimulating hormone (FSH) and luteinizing hormone (LH) (produced in the pituitary gland), and estrogen and progesterone (from the ovaries).

A monthly cycle begins when the pituitary gland in your brain secretes FSH, which triggers the follicles (the eggs in their sacs) to produce estradiol (the body's natural estrogen). When the estrogen in your body peaks, the hypothalamus lets the pituitary know it's time to cut off the FSH and instead release a burst of LH. This triggers the release of an egg from a follicle in one of the ovaries—also known as *ovulation*—which will probably occur more than 500 times in your life.

The estradiol also triggers your uterus lining to thicken in anticipation of receiving a fertilized egg. Once ovulation has occurred, the follicle produces progesterone in addition to estrogen. If the egg isn't fertilized, progesterone levels drop and the uterine lining sheds and bleeds.

As you age, your store of eggs gradually diminishes, and the estrogen-secreting layer of cells becomes less responsive to the signals from the brain. Some months you won't ovulate at all, which means you don't produce any estrogen or progesterone. The result: you skip a period.

Some women in this situation have longer periods with heavy flow (if you still have enough estrogen to thicken the uterine wall, you may experience heavy bleeding when progesterone *is* finally produced). Others find they have shorter cycles and hardly any bleeding. Some have a combination of the two, and others will begin to miss periods completely. During this time, you also will experience a decrease in your ability to become pregnant.

Eight out of every hundred women stop menstruating before age 40. At the other end of the spectrum, five out of every hundred continue to have periods until they are almost 60.

As we've seen, by the time you reach your late 30s or 40s your ovaries begin to shut down, producing less estrogen and progesterone and releasing eggs less often. The gradual decline of estrogen causes a wide variety of changes in tissues that respond to estrogen—vagina, vulva, uterus, bladder, urethra, breasts, bones, heart, blood vessels, brain, skin, hair, and mucous membranes. You may notice that you get more colds and flu. That's because almost all tissues in your body have estrogen receptors; when the level drops, they may not function as well. Over the long run, the lack of estrogen can make you more vulnerable to osteoporosis (which can begin in the 40s) and heart disease.

As the levels of hormones in your body fall, you will begin to experience the symptoms of perimenopause. In fact, some women find that the very worst symptoms of the entire menopausal transition occur during the perimenopausal phase according to Gail Sheehy, author of *The Silent Passage.*

It's important to remember that perimenopause can be triggered not just by age but also by smoking, tubal ligation, hysterectomy, damaged reproductive organs, being underweight, or from a severely restricted diet.

When Will Perimenopause Arrive?

Unfortunately, there's no easy way to predict when you will enter the perimenopause years. There's no mathematical formula to figure out when your ovaries will begin to scale back, but you can get some general idea based on your family history, body type, and lifestyle.

First of all, there is no link between the age when you started menstruating and the age when you will stop. It is true that you will likely enter menopause at about the same age as your mother—but if your mother had a hysterectomy, as did many women of that generation, you may never know when she would have naturally entered menopause.

However, it's also true that the hormonal situation for many women today may be profoundly different from the experience of our ancestors. Because these women of long ago got married fairly soon after puberty and spent much of their lives either pregnant or nursing, they had many fewer periods than we have had today. This means that their lifetime exposure to estrogen was actually far lower than ours. How this difference in long-term exposure to hormones will affect the age at which modern women enter perimenopause is not fully understood.

On average, menopause begins at 51. If you want to have an idea when you may enter perimenopause, read the following conditional statements, and work backward or forward from that age to estimate when you will experience menopause.

Your menopause may be *earlier* than average (that is, age 51) if you:

- are thin or small boned

- have never had children

- don't smoke

- live at a high altitude

- have eaten poorly throughout your life

- have a higher standard of living

- have had a hysterectomy or tubal ligation (even if your ovaries aren't removed, a woman whose uterus has been removed appears to enter menopause a few years earlier than otherwise)

- have shorter-than-average cycles (less than 25 days)

- have had several abortions

Your menopause may be *later* than average if you:

- are heavy or big boned

- have had several children (each child you've had will delay the onset of menopause by about five months)

- smoke

- live at sea level

- have had diabetes, cancer of the breast or uterus, or uterine fibroid tumors

- have a lower standard of living

- had your first child after age 40

- have taken birth control pills for many years

PMS and Perimenopause

Because so many of the symptoms of perimenopause seem to mimic those of premenstrual syndrome (PMS), some women find it hard to tell the difference. The seven million women with PMS notice that symptoms usually begin either with the first period or after the first pregnancy. Some physicians believe that an attack of PMS that suddenly appears in your 30s may not be PMS at all, but very early signs of perimenopause. Certainly some of the symptoms—moodiness, irritability, breast tenderness, headaches—are the same for both problems.

There is no agreement as to whether women with significant PMS that begins in the teenage years will go on to develop many problems in perimenopause. Likewise, there doesn't appear to be a correlation between severity of PMS and severity of perimenopause symptoms.

If you suspect you have PMS and not perimenopause, it helps to keep a diary of symptoms. Note the date when symptoms begin and any changes in symptoms. PMS symptoms tend to be cyclical; perimenopause symptoms are not. Keeping a diary will help to chart when these symptoms occur and what, if anything, appears to set them off.

What's Next?

In the next chapter you'll learn about all the symptoms of perimenopause along with a variety of lifestyle changes you can make to ease your symptoms right now. If these lifestyle changes don't help, the next step may be to try one of a variety of "alternative" treatments—meditation, yoga, herbs, plant estrogens, biofeedback, acupuncture, and so on. These alternative methods are described in Chapter 5. If these other remedies don't work, and your physician agrees that you might want to consider hormone replacement, there's a full discussion of the pros and cons in Chapter 6.

2 Symptoms of Perimenopause

The most common symptom of early menopause is a change in your menstrual cycle, but there are many other symptoms of early menopause as well. The most common of these are hot flashes, insomnia, mood swings, memory or concentration problems, and vaginal dryness.

But according to experts, these common symptoms may not be the only problems you encounter. Perimenopause can also affect your everyday life and your relationship with your partner and your children because of poor communication about the symptoms you're having. Although many women complain of hot flashes, depression, mood swings, and night sweats, their partners often are not aware of these problems. Instead of their partners, many women confide in their women friends and physicians for emotional support during perimenopause. If you don't confide in your partner, the reasons behind your mood swings and other symptoms may be misunderstood. Indeed, one nationwide survey found that 35 percent of women reported that, as they entered menopause, they argued more with their families.

If you have a couple of the following symptoms, you may want to contact your doctor. For many of these symptoms, the discussion includes a "what you can do" section to offer suggestions on lifestyle changes that may help you deal with particular problems. For the most part, these tips involve things you can do on your own to help take control of your own symptoms. If you feel you need more help in controlling the symptoms but you're not ready for hormone replacement, or your doctor is reluctant to prescribe hormones if you're still menstruating, Chapter 5 discusses some alternative ways of regulating symptoms. Standard hormone replacement therapy is discussed in Chapter 6.

Bleeding (heavy)

Although there is a wide variation in the length of menstrual cycles from woman to woman, as you enter early menopause your own cycles will become more irregular or farther apart. They may be heavier or lighter in flow. Some women notice a combination of all three symptoms that vary from month to month.

Shorter cycles can be an indication that you aren't ovulating anymore. Ovulation usually occurs in the middle of a menstrual cycle; as the amount of estrogen in your body drops, the number of days before you reach the midpoint of your cycle will decrease. At the same time as the amount of progesterone drops, the number of days *after* the cycle midpoint varies. Low levels of both hormones will have a strong effect on your cycle.

Missed periods are not uncommon because in some months you won't ovulate; this means you won't produce progesterone and you won't shed your uterine lining. You can tell the difference between a missed period and a pregnancy by the presence of other symptoms. A missed period that occurs along with dryness of the vagina and hot flashes is most likely related to perimenopause. A missed period together with nausea, fatigue, and breast tenderness may be pregnancy. If you have any doubts, see your doctor. Although you could take a home pregnancy test, older women may find that their fluctuating hormones are more likely to cause a false positive on such a test.

If you notice heavy bleeding or long intervals of spotting, or you have gone more than two months without a period, you should talk to your doctor. These symptoms—especially heavy bleeding—may be due to more serious problems such as polyps, fibroid tumors, or cancer.

Almost a fourth of all hysterectomies in the United States are performed in an effort to control prolonged abnormal bleeding. If the only reason you are having problems with bleeding is due to perimenopausal hormone changes, hormone replacement therapy may make a hysterectomy unnecessary. Keep in mind that this abnormal bleeding will stop once menopause is complete. Before agreeing to a hysterectomy, get a second and third opinion.

If your bleeding is related to fibroids, a hysterectomy may be a wise choice if there is painful pressure on your rectum or bladder and when other treatments, such as D&C (dilation and curettage) or hormonal tablets, haven't helped the problem. You may need a hysterectomy for rapidly growing fibroids because they are occasionally malignant. Fibroid growth can be measured by ultrasound; an endometrial biopsy can rule out the possibility of cancer.

What You Can Do

It is possible to help control heavy bleeding by making some lifestyle changes.

- Avoid hot baths or showers—remember that heat dilates blood vessels, which can increase your flow.

- Don't take aspirin. Aspirin is a "blood thinner," which means that it can increase your blood flow by interfering with the clotting ability of blood platelets.

- Avoid alcohol. When you drink a lot, fewer blood platelets form, which means your blood won't clot as well and you may experience a heavier flow during your periods.

- Exercise. Remember that exercising will lower the release of hormones FSH and LH, which will lower the amount of estrogen released by your ovaries.

CHECKUPS FOR WOMEN WITH HEAVY FLOW

If you are bleeding heavily and irregularly, you need to have your blood checked for signs of anemia. If the test reveals low levels of hemoglobin, eat more iron-rich foods and take iron supplements.

Heavy or irregular bleeding also can be caused by a dysfunctional thyroid gland. Have your thyroid checked for abnormally low or high levels of the thyroid hormone.

Bloated Feeling

Salt can increase the bloated feeling—not just salt you add to food, but also salt already present in prepared foods.

What You Can Do

- Use herbs and spices instead of salt.

- Avoid adding extra salt.

Breast Changes

It's quite common to experience changes in breast tenderness or fullness with the menstrual cycle and pregnancy; this also occurs during perimenopause. Breast tissue is very sensitive to estrogen and progesterone, even in amounts produced during a normal cycle.

Women undergoing hormone replacement therapy may also experience breast tenderness. This should diminish or become tolerable in a few weeks after beginning therapy; if it doesn't, you should check with your doctor.

Of course, any lumps or thickening that you may find in your breast at any time should be evaluated by your doctor, who may recommend a mammogram, depending on your family history.

Depression

Although a mild depression affects many women and may be related to many of the symptoms of perimenopause, experts no longer believe that depression is caused by the onset of perimenopausal symptoms.

Once called "involutional melancholia," it was described as a disorder that occurred during menopause characterized by worry, anxiety, agitation, and severe insomnia. This concept was eliminated from the American Psychiatric Association's bible of disorders, the *Diagnostic and Statistical Manual of Mental Disorders*, in 1980. Subsequent studies have failed to show any link between depression and menopause; women who do become depressed during this time don't appear to have symptoms of depression that are any different from younger women.

Of course, this doesn't mean you won't ever get depressed as you enter the perimenopause period. Inevitably, some women do become depressed—but not because of perimenopause itself. If you aren't sleeping well, perimenopause can disturb healthy sleep patterns; fatigue caused by interrupted sleep can make you feel depressed. But it's important to note the difference between symptom-related feelings of depression and emotional illness.

It's also true that if you are depressed, you might be more bothered by symptoms of perimenopause; women who are already depressed are more than twice as likely to see a doctor to complain about hot flashes, cold sweats, and irregular periods. If you are feeling depressed, you need to talk to a mental health care expert about treatment for depression.

Fatigue

Another very common symptom is a feeling of exhaustion. It's not surprising that if you're struggling with insomnia or you're up all night with hot flashes, you're going to be tired during the day. That nagging feeling of exhaustion is usually a combination of physical and emotional elements.

What You Can Do

- It may seem like a contradiction in terms, but exercise is one of the best ways to combat fatigue. When you're feeling tired, don't flop on the couch and turn on the TV—go out for a walk.

- Try anything aerobic to get your heart pumping; when your heart is working hard, that rush of adrenaline will trigger the release of endorphins, the chemical brain substances that naturally make you feel good.

- See Chapter 8 for more information on starting your own exercise program.

Hair Changes

As you enter perimenopause, you may notice the appearance of darker hair on your face. As the level of estrogen drops, our male hormones (androgens) are no longer kept in "balance" by the estrogen. As a result, hair may begin to grow in response to the androgen that was always present in your body but that didn't cause the hair to grow before because estrogen was present. You may notice hair appearing in a more typically "masculine" pattern—on upper lip, chin, and cheeks. Women undergoing HRT will notice this hair growth stopping, although the hair already present on your face won't go away.

At the same time you may notice you're losing hair on your head, arms, legs, and genital area. This is because the tissue that supports the hair follicles tends to diminish as we get older—the skin gets thinner and drier, and the fat and muscle under the skin shrinks. If you are upset about significant hair loss—female baldness is rare but not unheard of—you can discuss the problem with a dermatologist or gynecologist, who may be able to help.

Headaches

Fluctuating levels of estrogen can cause headaches, especially if you were prone to premenstrual migraines before perimenopause. In addition, if you are taking hormone replacement therapy, you may experience intense headaches at first in response to the initial boost in hormones.

What You Can Do

- Avoid anything that triggered headaches before you entered perimenopause—certain types of food, caffeine, alcohol, stress.
- Regular exercise or biofeedback may help.
- Your doctor may prescribe pain medication if you are having severe headaches.
- If you are on HRT and you know you tend to get headaches anyway, you can choose the patch instead of a pill; patches provide a more constant absorption of hormone, which can lessen the risk of headaches.

Heart Palpitations

The rapid, out-of-control sensation of heart palpitations is a fairly common symptom of perimenopause, caused by a vasomotor response in the brain. However, it's important to realize they can also be caused by a variety of other factors, including too much caffeine or nicotine—or a heart condition. You need to discuss any heart palpitations with your physician.

Hot Flashes and Night Sweats

The second most common symptom of perimenopause is hot flashes. According to a 1991 Gallup survey, 87 percent of perimenopausal women report they have experienced hot flashes, and more than half say they also experience night sweats. About half of women, according to another study, experience hot flashes while they are still menstruating regularly.

Although some women may notice only an occasional hot flash that prompts them to remove a sweater or briefly fan themselves, other women wake in the middle of the night drenched in sweat, with soaking sheets.

Others find it difficult to function in their daily lives because they are so uncomfortable.

Your face may suddenly feel flushed or blotchy; sweat may roll off your body, and your skin may feel hot to the touch. Most of the time the feeling of heat begins just above your waist, spreading quickly to the chest, back, neck, face, and scalp. The sensations of searing heat may last anywhere from a few seconds to an hour, either once or twice a day or as often as 40 or 50 times daily. Although hot flashes usually only occur for about a year—one of the most transitory of all the perimenopause symptoms—some women struggle with them for up to five years. Most of the time they occur when you're sitting still or when you're asleep, but they can be triggered as well by exercise, eating spicy food, or drinking a hot beverage.

Cause

The precise mechanism behind hot flashes is not completely understood, but they are believed to be related to changes in the hypothalamus as you experience estrogen withdrawal and declining hormone levels.

The hypothalamus—the body's "temperature" gland—contains temperature-sensitive brain cells that step up their activity when you get too hot or cold. When you get too warm, your hypothalamus sends a chemical message that triggers your blood vessels to dilate, to release excess heat. The hypothalamus tells your sweat glands just under the skin to perspire to help cool you off. If your brain senses your body is too cold, it constricts blood vessels to keep heat from escaping, and sets off the shivering response to boost metabolism.

A hot flash occurs when your hypothalamus gets confused. For some reason, it starts to trigger the cooling response at the wrong time because it senses the body is hotter than it really is, triggering all the mechanisms of your body to cool you off. When you first begin the flash, your skin gets cold and clammy; your blood vessels dilate, and your heart rate speeds up. Skin temperature may rise by up to eight degrees Fahrenheit, and you begin to sweat. In other words—you start experiencing a hot flash.

As a result of these efforts, your core body temperature drops within five to nine minutes after the flash begins. When your core temperature drops, your blood vessels constrict, metabolism increases, and you start to shiver.

Doctors believe estrogen plays a role in hot flashes because they begin as estrogen levels drop—and they begin abruptly when ovaries are removed. (Studies have shown that the more abruptly a woman's estrogen levels fall, the more severe the hot flashes will be.) This is why women who have had their ovaries removed experience much more severe hot flashes than those whose ovaries are intact. This is also why thin women have stronger hot flashes—fat cells produce estrogen even after menopause is complete.

The reason why scientists are certain that estrogen is linked to hot flashes is that when these women are given estrogen replacement, hot flashes stop. But the exact interaction between estrogen and the brain remains unclear because once you have been in menopause for some time your estrogen levels remain low, but you don't continue to have hot flashes. Hot flashes have also been reported during pregnancy when estrogen levels are high. For this reason, experts suspect hot flashes are more likely the result of estrogen *withdrawal,* and not *low* estrogen levels.

Studies suggest that estrogen does increase the activity of brain cells sensitive to heat, and decreases the activity of brain cells sensitive to cold.

It's probably true that estrogen doesn't act alone. Other hormones and various brain chemicals may also be involved. Progesterone, for example, appears to rise during the second half of your cycle, raising your body temperature and making you feel warmer. And several types of neurotransmitters are intimately related to the functioning of your hypothalamus.

The episodes are most likely to accompany PMS or occur during missed cycles. Some women also notice feelings of tingling, throbbing, or dizziness as they feel the first flush of heat. In addition, more than 68 percent of women note that they also experience night sweats.

Some women are more affected by hot flashes than others because their level of estrogen doesn't drop slowly and evenly, but fluctuates wildly. As the body tries to repeatedly adjust, the hot flashes become stronger and more frequent.

Although you may not experience hot flashes, you may experience night sweats caused by the same vasomotor symptoms that cause hot flashes. Night sweating is a common problem that often follows hot flashes. When you're in bed, you'll feel especially hot because your body underneath the covers is warmer at night, and because if you're asleep you won't be able to do anything to head off the hot flash.

What You Can Do

- Ten minutes of slow, deep abdominal breathing (six to eight breaths per minute) every morning and night can lower hot flashes by 40 percent, according to one study.

- Exercise. Studies show that hot flashes are half as common in women who are physically active (aerobic activity) as in those who are sedentary.

- Stop smoking. Smoking constricts blood vessels, which can intensify a hot flash.

- Choose natural fabrics. Cotton and other nonsynthetic fabrics tend to breathe and don't trap perspiration. If you have night sweats, cotton sheets and short-sleeve night clothes with a V neck are good choices.

- Avoid foods that seem to bring on a hot flash (sugar, coffee, alcohol, spicy foods, teas, colas, chocolate, salt, hot soups, or hot drinks).

- Keep track of your hot flashes. If you find a pattern, you may be able to manage the symptoms because you know when to expect them.

- Sip a cold drink. Keep a thermos of cold juice or water nearby.

- Take a cold shower or splash cold water on your wrists or face. Use an air conditioner in your bedroom, and buy a portable fan to carry in your purse.

- Suck on a piece of hard candy; some women say that this can head off a hot flash or moderate a strong hot flash.

- Ginseng is a popular remedy for night sweats in doses of 1,000 mg daily. Ginseng is also a stimulant, however; overdoses can lead to insomnia and anxiety.

Insomnia

About two in ten women experience "menopause insomnia," the inability to fall asleep during perimenopause. Experts believe the sleep problems are due to falling levels of estrogen. Hot flashes and night sweats can cause chronic sleep deprivation, which can make you even more irritable, moody, depressed, or forgetful.

What You Can Do

- At bedtime drink a glass of warm milk, take a hot bath, listen to soft music, or read. Don't pay bills, exercise, or watch an exciting movie and then try to fall asleep.

- Avoid caffeine, chocolate, and spicy food late at night. Drink your last cup of coffee no later than 4 P.M.

- Exercise—but avoid working out any later than two hours before bedtime, or your heightened metabolism may block sleep.

- Go to bed the same time each night.

- Try relaxation: because insomnia may be related to stress, you may find relief through meditation, yoga, prayer, or progressive relaxation. (See details in Chapter 8.)

- Avoid alcohol; although you may have been able to tolerate alcohol in the past, your present insomnia may be alcohol related. Cut back and see. Alcohol can make you wake up within a few hours of going to sleep, and it keeps you from reaching a deep sleep.

- Stop smoking.

- Cut back on some types of antihistamines; they may be related to insomnia, even if you've never had a problem with them in the past.

- Don't eat a big meal right before bed, and keep your bedroom cool and dark.

- Use cotton sheets (you'll sweat less).

- If all else fails, you may want to try biofeedback or a sleep disorders clinic.

Irritability and Mood Swings

You're standing at the counter, and the pharmacist tells you she's all out of your favorite brand of panty hose. You burst into tears. No, you're not losing your mind and becoming emotionally unbalanced.

At least 60 percent women report they have experienced anxiety, irritability, or nervousness during perimenopause, and nearly 58 percent say they have experienced mood swings or some depression. As your hormones fluctuate, it's perfectly normal to feel tense and irritable and cry easily. Estrogen and progesterone affect chemicals in the brain that control sleep, pain perception, and a wide variety of emotions, diminishing your ability to cope with problems that you normally handle with ease.

If you're stressed out in addition to the symptoms of perimenopause, this will only make your feelings of tension or irritability worse.

What You Can Do

- Eat a well-balanced diet rich in fruits and vegetables.

- Get plenty of exercise.

- Reduce stress; meditation has been shown to help ease perimenopausal symptoms.

- Join a support group of perimenopausal women.

Sexual Disinterest

"I used to have a wonderful sexual relationship with my husband," Shelly commented. "But lately, I find myself waiting until I'm sure he's asleep before I go to bed. I just don't care about sex anymore. What's wrong with me?"

Declining levels of estrogen can have a direct effect on your libido. Lower estrogen levels also can make your genitals less sensitive and make sex painful due to dry vaginal tissues. Of course, it's also possible that your loss of interest in sex is related to something else—exhaustion from lack of sleep, or depression, or PMS.

However, the male sex hormone testosterone is probably more responsible for maintaining sexual desire than estrogen. High levels of the male hormone have been linked to desire and sexual fantasies among women past menopause and in women who take testosterone supplements. Although total testosterone levels do decline somewhat as you enter perimenopause, levels of free testosterone—which is more biologically active—remain unchanged.

What You Can Do

- Keep having sex. The less often you have sex, the less you may begin to enjoy it.

- You can use commercial lubricants, or you can try vitamin E oil, egg white, or yogurt (this can also help control common yeast infections in the vagina).

- Take more time to make love.

- Experiment—try new things, as long as they aren't emotionally uncomfortable for you or your partner.

- Take a mini-vacation, even if it's just a hotel room in your own town. Get a sitter and go out to dinner; try a Jacuzzi.

Thinking and Memory Problems

There haven't been very many studies done on the effect of perimenopause and short-term memory, but many women insist that there appears to be a problem. Some of the most disturbing symptoms of perimenopause are the mental problems that can occur, including disorientation, concentration problems, and memory loss.

"I have trouble remembering which is the hot faucet and which is the cold faucet," commented one woman. "That's not something I ever had a problem with before—but I have to stop and *think* about which is which."

Women say that the memory loss begins with difficulty in concentrating, or forgetting where you put things. The problems with mental acuity may well be linked to the dropping estrogen level, according to researchers. The brain, like the uterus and breasts, contains estrogen receptors (sites where hormones can affect cells). In one study at Rockefeller University, researchers found that lower estrogen levels in lab animals may reduce the number of connections between brain cells, leading to problems of concentration and memory. Related studies found that lower estrogen levels may lead to a drop in the brain chemical serotonin, a neurotransmitter related to mood and depression.

The more abrupt your estrogen withdrawal, the more pronounced the symptoms. This is why women recovering from surgery or chemotherapy may experience a particular memory problem.

Of course, some problems with memory and concentration are an inevitable part of aging for men and women. But there is a difference between the age-related problem of *retrieving* information you have stored in your memory banks and perimenopause-related forgetfulness. If your short-term memory is dramatically worse—not only can't you remember where you parked your car, but you have no recollection of even driving into the parking garage—your symptoms may be linked to estrogen withdrawal. Moreover, memory and concentration may be made worse if you also have problems in getting to sleep at night.

Estrogen therapy was found to improve memory in a study in Canada of 72-year-old women taking estrogen and another group not taking the hormone. The women taking estrogen performed better in several memory tests than did the women not on estrogen. The first study showing that estrogen could improve memory loss was published in 1954; since then, other studies have shown that HRT can significantly improve functioning in postmenopausal women diagnosed with Alzheimer's disease. Postmenopausal women who receive HRT are up to 60 percent less likely to develop Alzheimer's disease.

What You Can Do

- Make lists and notes for yourself.

- Carry a tiny battery-powered, microchip "note recorder" to keep track of appointments, notes to yourself, and other things you need to remember.

- Pay attention. Many memory lapses occur because we are distracted, stressed, or thinking of something else when we put keys down or park the car.

- Get enough sleep if you want to boost your concentration the next day.

- Exercise your brain: take up new hobbies, learn a foreign language or chess, work on your computer skills. "Use it or lose it" doesn't apply just to sex.

Urinary Changes

"I don't know what's happening lately," complains Ann, 43, "but whenever I sneeze, some urine leaks into my underwear!"

Many women report changes in urination beginning with perimenopause. You may find yourself in Ann's shoes, facing stress incontinence—the inability to hold in your urine during moments of stress, such as when you sneeze, laugh, or run. Or you may feel as if you are going to the bathroom all the time. Other women complain that the urge to urinate is so strong they can barely restrain it until they reach a bathroom. When you do urinate, you may find it has become painful.

Losing control during times of stress is caused by loosening muscles around the bladder and urethra. As the vaginal wall weakens as a result of estrogen depletion, it can no longer support the bladder, which can drop out of place. Without the support of the vaginal wall and other muscles, even the tiniest pressure of a sneeze or a cough can lead to a small loss of urine. Women who have had hysterectomies sometimes experience incontinence because the missing uterus has left the bladder and urethra without support, and occasionally the surgery itself can damage urinary tissues.

Moreover, lower estrogen levels can lead to changes in the urethra much like those that occur in the vagina, setting off or worsening incontinence problems.

Urinary infections (which can cause an urge to urinate, frequent urination, or pain) are also due to a drop in estrogen. The urethra has estrogen receptors, and without the hormone it can atrophy in the same way as the vagina. As the urethral walls become thinner and weaker, they are more prone to develop infections.

You may experience more urinary tract infections because the urethra and bladder tissue become thinner and less elastic. This makes these tissues more vulnerable to infection. Because repeated infections may endanger your kidneys or bladder, you should contact a doctor at the first sign of a urinary tract infection.

KEGEL EXERCISES

Kegel exercises can help with bladder control, tightening and toning the vaginal area. Kegel exercises (named for Dr. Arnold Kegel, a UCLA surgeon who developed them in the 1950s) can be done in one of two ways. In either case, try to do at least ten sets of 20 each day:

1. Contract your vaginal muscles as if you were trying to stop yourself from urinating.

2. Hold for a count of five; relax for a count of five; repeat this sequence 20 times.

Pelvic relaxation that is too severe to respond to Kegels or HRT (see Chapter 4) may require surgical intervention. However, surgery should be a last resort. Be sure to have your doctor assess your bladder function with a cystometrogram before agreeing to surgery.

What You Can Do

- If you don't want to try Kegels, you may be interested in pelvic training weights, a set of weights that look like small cones with attached strings, ranging from 20 to 70 grams. You begin by inserting the smallest weight into the vagina, wearing it for 10 to 15 minutes twice a day. Your circumvaginal muscles must hold the weight in the vagina (otherwise, it falls out). When you can hold the weight in place even when coughing, you graduate to the next larger weight.

- Lose weight; extra weight may put too much stress on the bladder and urethra, causing them to sag and leak.

- Some drugs (such as antihistamines and tranquilizers) can aggravate bladder control problems.

- Some foods or beverages (spicy foods or citrus beverages) can irritate the bladder and worsen leakage. Cut back or eliminate caffeine and alcohol for the same reason.

- Exercise to strengthen your abdomen and pelvic muscles.

- To prevent infections, drink plenty of fluids, urinate completely, and don't hold your urine; always wipe front to back; change tampons or pads regularly; ask your doctor to test the acid-base balance of your vagina (if the level is above 4.5, consider using an estrogen cream). Studies show that drinking two eight-ounce glasses of cranberry juice a day can help prevent urinary infections.

Vaginal Dryness

You may notice vaginal dryness during perimenopause, which can be severe enough to make intercourse uncomfortable. It may not be something that you discuss with your friends or your partner, but it is very common.

The vagina is a five-inch-long tunnel of muscle lined with moist skin that can stretch during intercourse and expand a great deal during childbirth. The vagina produces a clear acidic discharge that helps protect against infections; when you become sexually aroused, the vagina becomes lubricated in preparation for sexual activity.

As you enter perimenopause, estrogen levels fall and your vaginal walls become drier and thinner. This dryness is your body's response to the declining level of estrogen; the vaginal secretions also become less acidic. This opens the way for more vaginal infections. As estrogen levels drop, your vaginal lining gets thinner and less elastic; eventually, the vagina itself may become shorter and narrower. If untreated, the vagina can actually atrophy.

This lack of lubrication can make sex uncomfortable—even painful. In severe cases the vaginal walls can actually tear and bleed.

What You Can Do

- Before having sex, smear a few teaspoons of a water-soluble jelly (such as K-Y or Astroglide) on the outside of your vagina, and a little bit on the inside. Water-based lubricants are better than oil-based ones because they are less likely to cause infection. You should use a jelly specifically made for use during sex. Don't use petroleum jelly; it can break down the latex of a condom, increasing your vulnerability to sexually transmitted diseases. Astroglide is a light lubricant that doesn't have any medicinal taste or smell; it is applied right before intercourse.

- Alternatively, you could try a vaginal moisturizer (such as Replens) rather than a lubricant, which can be applied hours before intercourse. These moisturizers claim to replenish vaginal moisture when used regularly. To use, insert the applicator into the vagina three or four times a week so that it coats the surface of the vagina and moisturizes the tissues.

- Drink plenty of water; you can also drink fruit or vegetable juices or herbal teas. (Coffee and alcohol will dehydrate you, so you might want to avoid them.)

- Stimulate the vaginal area to boost blood flow and improve lubrication; have regular intercourse or masturbate regularly.

- Avoid douches, perfumed toilet paper, bath bubbles, soaps, or oils that can dry or irritate your vagina.

- Don't become anxious, because tension can lead to painful intercourse.

- Avoid antihistamines and other drugs that cause dryness.

- Engage in longer foreplay so your body has time to release its own lubricants. By the time you reach your mid-50s, you will need longer stimulation to become fully lubricated.

- Don't wear tight pants or underpants that don't have a cotton lining.

Weight Gain

As you approach perimenopause, you may be alarmed as you see your body change. Many women begin to put on weight, and start to notice areas of fat that seem to appear out of nowhere. As you age, more of what you're eating turns to fat instead of muscle. And as your body fat realigns, it can make you appear heavier even if you haven't gained a pound.

Of course, it's not impossible to have a good body after the age of 40 or 50—but you may have to work at it a bit harder. You also may not be able to eat quite the same fat-loaded foods you did before.

What You Can Do

- Follow sensible, good eating habits (see Chapter 8).

- If you haven't already, begin an exercise routine and stick with it— even if it's just a walk around the block.

- See Chapter 8 to set up your own exercise plan.

Other Physical Symptoms

A few women report a whole menagerie of other symptoms, such as food cravings, but many of these are really secondary effects of the primary symptoms. For example, painful intercourse is really the result of drying and thinning of vaginal tissue.

What's Next?

Clearly, the best way to ease your transition through perimenopause is to be prepared for it. Because knowledge is power, the more you know about your physical condition, the better you will be able to handle it.

It won't be surprising to many women that experts disagree on the best ways to treat the symptoms of perimenopause. Opinions vary a great deal about whether or not to treat these women, how, and when to do so. Experts do agree that this is the best time to start paying attention to your total health and to take steps that will affect your well-being in the years to come. In the next chapter you'll learn about how to determine if you are, in fact, experiencing perimenopausal symptoms.

3

How to Tell If You're in Early Menopause (Diagnosis)

The perimenopause years are typically a time of transition for many women. Even as your body is trying to cope with a dramatic readjustment and rebalancing of your reproductive organs, your entry into midlife means you may be dealing with a host of midlife changes, including maturing children, job changes, stress, or problems with your own aging parents.

Sharon, 43, was facing the fact that her only daughter was leaving for college this fall. Finally giving up on her job after many years, she was launching her own consulting business. At the same time, she was facing the necessity of putting her father in a nursing home following the death of her mother. She often felt overwhelmed, anxious, and moody. Sometimes it seemed as if her mind was in a fog, and she was often tired and depressed. All these symptoms could be related to the stress of her midlife transition—but they could also be traced to an early menopause.

How can you tell whether your symptoms are simply the result of psychological issues, or whether they are caused by physical changes in your body? A simple test to determine the onset of perimenopause would be handy, but none exists. Although the first major study of women who are undergoing the midlife transition is currently going on, data won't be available for another year or two.

FSH Test

Some doctors believe that the FSH test can determine whether or not you are in menopause, but in reality it's not quite that simple. The FSH test is a measure of the level of follicle-stimulating hormone in your blood. As your estrogen level drops, your pituitary and hypothalamus secrete more FSH in response to the low levels of estrogen, desperately trying to stimulate sluggish estrogen-producing cells to release an egg from your ovaries. The ovaries produce a burst of estrogen, followed by ovulation. If you do ovulate, your progesterone will rise; when your period does come, it will tend to be very heavy because of the extra estrogen.

This pattern of fluctuation is very typical of perimenopause; if your estrogen levels are high and your progesterone is low, you may have the mood swings, irritability, and other symptoms characteristic of PMS. When your hormone levels shift and your estrogen level falls, you experience hot flashes. Then your levels may even out for a time until the next fluctuation. It is this ebb and flow of estrogen—*not* the low levels of estrogen alone—that causes your symptoms of perimenopause. Although it's true that FSH levels rise steadily as you age, women have varying patterns of FSH levels and menopause symptoms.

Simply measuring your FSH level at any one point in time will only give you a picture of what is going on in your body at that particular moment. It won't tell you reliably whether or not you are perimenopausal because your FSH levels are fluctuating just as your estrogen does.

In one recent study scientists discovered that it is possible for some women to keep on menstruating with high levels of FSH, even as other women have high levels of FSH and low levels of estrogen. Other women experienced wild fluctuations of FSH, with readings typical of post-menopause one month and levels that plummeted to perimenopausal levels the next.

If it has been at least three months since your last period, a test of your FSH level might be a bit more helpful in determining whether or not you have finally entered menopause—but even this is no guarantee. It's possible to stop having periods for several months, and then abruptly begin bleeding again. In fact, one study found that this is exactly what happened to about 20 percent of women who had apparently stopped having their periods.

However, if your periods have slowed down and you haven't had a period in about three months, it may be possible to get a more accurate reading via the FSH test. At this point an FSH level of 20 or more miu/ml (milli international units per milliliter) indicates that perimenopause has started. On the other hand, the average FSH for a young menstruating woman is less than 5 miu/ml. Once the FSH level exceeds 20 miu/ml, 80 percent of women will experience menopause within a year. When the FSH level reaches 40 miu/ml, menopause is said to be complete.

Most doctors believe that the FSH test alone can't be used as proof that you've entered perimenopause, and in any case, it doesn't give you the information you need to manage this change.

Test All Hormones

Instead of just a test to measure the amount of FSH, insist that you have a test that also checks the levels of estrogen, progesterone, testosterone, and other hormones at mid-cycle. Contrary to popular belief, estrogen isn't the only hormone that changes during perimenopause.

The only true marker of perimenopause is having irregular periods—spotting, lengthened or shortened cycles, heavy bleeding, and cramps. However, because abnormal bleeding (especially abnormally heavy bleeding) can be caused by fibroids, hormone imbalances, and cancer, it's imperative to get checked out by a doctor if you're experiencing irregular bleeding.

Hot flashes and night sweats are common perimenopausal symptoms, but they also accompany the postpartum period. Moodiness and cramps can be perimenopausal, but they may also be due to premenstrual syndrome. Because so many of the symptoms of perimenopause can be confused with other conditions, doctors don't always correctly diagnose a woman—especially one they think is too young to be approaching menopause.

What's Next?

In the next chapter you'll learn whether or not you need a specialist to help you manage your perimenopausal transition and how to find one if you do. You'll learn the questions to ask, where to find the professional you want, and how to choose the best person to join your health care team.

4

Getting Help: Finding the Right Doctor

Jennifer, 42, was having a lot of trouble with memory problems, vaginal dryness, and hot flashes. "My doctor at the HMO just didn't seem to *hear* me," she complained. "He was willing to put me on hormones, but I just wanted to talk to someone who I thought would really listen to me."

Jennifer referred herself to a reproductive endocrinologist, who counseled her to avoid HRT for the moment and try to deal with her vaginal dryness with a vaginal hormone cream. "I finally found someone who listened to my complaints without making me feel like I was just being a stereotypical whining woman," she explained.

Types of Traditional Physicians

- **family practitioner** A physician who provides comprehensive medical care for everyone in the family, treating all problems and making referrals to specialists as necessary.

- **gynecologist** A physician who specializes in diagnosing and treating problems of the female reproductive tract, including problems relating to menstruation and perimenopause. A gynecologist also offers advice on contraception and can treat infertility. Many gynecologists are also obstetricians. A woman should see a gynecologist every one to three years from the time she begins menstruating, for a pelvic exam and a cervical smear (Pap test).

- **internist** A specialist in the diagnosis and treatment of adult diseases, especially those related to the internal organs. Internists often provide primary care.

- **reproductive endocrinologist** An endocrinologist who specializes in problems involving reproductive hormones, such as the problems a woman faces during perimenopause.

- **specialist in hormone replacement therapy** A provider with this specialty may well place emphasis on treating your symptoms with HRT and may not include other alternative or less-intensive treatment regimens.

- **specialist in menopause** A menopause specialist can tailor your health care and may or may not include HRT. Alternatives could include nutrition, herbs, vitamins, exercise, and preventive care.

How to Choose a Specialist

Many women have tended to rely on their gynecologist for all their health care needs. As you age, however, and your health care concerns broaden, you may want to find an internist or family care physician. If you choose a family care physician or internist for your gynecological care as well, you'll need to be sure this specialist also performs an annual pelvic exam and Pap smear.

As you enter perimenopause, you may prefer to locate a doctor who is an expert in the field of menopause. A reproductive endocrinologist is a specialist who might be a good choice if you have severe symptoms during perimenopause.

If you're faced with perimenopause symptoms, you should seek help from a health care provider trained in the treatment of midlife issues, including menopause. But should that be an internist, a gynecologist, or a reproductive endocrinologist? Or maybe a nurse practitioner, acupuncturist, or naturopath would be more in tune with your needs.

There is a wide range of specialists, in addition to internists or family physicians, from whom to choose. You'll want to find someone you can work with, someone who won't dismiss your complaints and overlook symptoms—someone you can work with as a team. It's essential that you are to be able to trust your health care provider and can feel comfortable with that person.

It's important to know which specialist to choose, because many symptoms of other diseases may masquerade as perimenopause. This is what happened to Bonnie, who at age 38 began to notice physical and emotional changes that were upsetting to her. She seemed to have trouble concentrating; her moods became erratic. Ordinarily an even-tempered, calm individual, she began to feel as if she were going to explode. Miserable with her symptoms, she trooped from doctor to doctor in a vain attempt at uncovering the reason behind her problems.

None of the doctors could find a medical reason for the symptoms, and one went so far as to recommend a psychiatrist, believing that her problems were "all in your head." Finally, at age 41, she was diagnosed as perimenopausal by a gynecologist. After she had taken birth control pills for a few months, her mood changes, night sweats, and mental fogginess disappeared.

Menopause Specialists

Sometimes you need more specialized care than you feel you're getting with your regular family doctor, internist, or gynecologist. If this is the case, you may be referred to a reproductive endocrinologist. A reproductive endocrinologist can be of special help if you are perimenopausal and trying to conceive, your symptoms are severe and aren't responding to traditional treatment, or you've had breast cancer or have close family members with the disease and you want someone with the latest information on HRT.

If you decide to find a specialist yourself without a referral, you can obtain a list of qualified reproductive endocrinologists from the American Fertility Society (see Appendix A).

Unless you live in a metropolitan area or near a large medical center, you may have to travel to find a good specialist, who will also tend to be expensive. However, it's possible to have most of your needs taken care of by your regular doctor and simply rely on the specialist for diagnosis and consultations. Most reproductive endocrinologists don't provide regular, ongoing gynecological care anyway, but will refer you back to your original doctor once your situation is stabilized.

TYPES OF ALTERNATIVE CARE PROVIDERS

* **acupuncturist** Acupuncture is a form of Chinese medicine involving the placement of needles along certain areas of the body to restore balance and ease symptoms. Many acupuncturists combine the use of acupuncture with Chinese herbs. In the United States acupuncture may be legally practiced by licensed physicians using disposable needles; acupuncture is a legal form of health care in at least 20 states, and some insurance companies will pay for the treatment. Those who live in states that license acupuncturists can find a list of certified practitioners at the state health or licensing department. A board-certified acupuncturist will use the initials "Dipl.Ac." after the name, which means "diplomate of acupuncture."

TYPES OF ALTERNATIVE CARE PROVIDERS *(continued)*

- **herbalist**   An herbalist is an expert in the use of herbs for the treatment of health problems, including perimenopausal symptoms; herbalists are not licensed in this country.

- **homeopathic doctor**   Homeopathic physicians use dilute solutions of naturally occurring substances that if given in full strength would provoke the same symptoms. Homeopathic practitioners are not licensed in homeopathy, but most experts are licensed in other health care specialties (M.D.s, chiropractors, naturopaths, acupuncturists, nurses, nurse practitioners, physicians' assistants, pharmacists, or dentists).

- **massage therapist**   Massage therapists perform a variety of massage techniques (including foot reflexology, shiatsu, and Swedish massage) in order to relieve stress and enhance circulation. You can find a certified massage therapist by contacting the American Massage Therapy Association.

- **naturopathic physician**   Practitioners of naturopathy follow a form of alternative medicine based on the idea that disease is caused by the accumulation of waste products and toxins in the body and that symptoms reflect the body's attempt to rid itself of these substances. Because the naturopathic philosophy includes the treatment of the "whole" woman, it can be a good choice for perimenopausal women looking for symptom relief. Naturopathic physicians are licensed in 13 states; you can obtain referrals from the American Association of Naturopathic Physicians.

- **nurse practitioner**   (nurse clinician) An RN who is trained to provide certain health services (including preventive care, monitoring of chronic conditions, physical exams, and health counseling) under the supervision of a physician. Many women's health centers include nurse practitioners on their staff.

Locating a Doctor

Once you've decided what kind of provider you'd like, you need to know how to go about finding one. You can start by asking friends or coworkers for recommendations, get a recommendation from your current family physician, or call your local hospital for a list of doctors affiliated with the institution.

Or you can find a doctor skilled in the treatment of perimenopause by contacting the North American Menopause Society (NAMS). They will send you a list of NAMS members, categorized by geographic location and specialty, that includes physicians, nurses, psychotherapists, social workers, and others who describe themselves as "menopause clinicians."

To ask for the list, write to NAMS, P.O. Box 94527, Cleveland, OH 44101; fax them at (216) 844-8708; or send an E-mail to *nams@apk.net.* By phone, call their 900 number at (900) 370-6267 (there is a charge for this call).

Next, you could check out the library resources, including *Compendium of Certified Medical Specialists* or *Directory of Medical Specialists*. These sources list physicians' credentials and whether or not they are board certified. (Board certified means a doctor has undergone extra training in that field, and has passed written and oral exams.)

Then narrow your choices based on which doctors have the most convenient location, whose office hours are most convenient, who accept your type of insurance, who are affiliated with a good local hospital, and whose office staff seem pleasant and well informed.

Next Stop: The Office Visit

Now that you have some names of potential doctors, it's time to schedule an office visit for the top two or three candidates. Talking on the phone to get some basic information is one thing, but you won't know how the doctor actually deals with you as a patient until you are sitting in the office.

Be sure to let the doctor know that you're there for an interview, and be prepared to pay the regular office visit fee. Make your final choice only after you've personally seen each doctor.

Your First Office Visit

If you want to get the most out of this visit, you need to do a little homework before you get to the office. You want to be prepared so you don't take up too much of the doctor's time—but you also need to have your questions answered. Being calm, serious, and organized will help.

Before you get to the doctor's office, it's a good idea to learn as much about perimenopause as you can. This way, you and your doctor can do the best job of exchanging information. Before you ever walk into the office of your new doctor, you may want to do the following things:

- If you're worried about having a long wait, call ahead a few hours before your appointment and see whether the office is running late.

- Have your relevant medical records from your previous doctor forwarded to the new office.

- Write down a list of questions you may have so you won't forget anything when you're with the doctor. (See the following section.)

- List the names and dosages of any drugs you take on a regular basis, and carry this information with you.

- Be prepared to discuss your symptoms confidently and seriously.

- Take an active, inquiring stance. If your doctor recommends any treatment, tests, or medication, you want to be sure you fully understand the reasons why, any potential side effects, and how the procedure will help.

Now review the following questions. Take this list along so you don't forget to ask everything you need to know.

Ten Questions to Ask the Doctor

1. Do you have specific training in menopause and aging?

2. Have you attended any menopause classes, courses, or workshops recently?

3. Do you offer any ongoing menopause support groups and/or classes? If not, can you recommend any workshops or classes?

4. Are you aware of, or open to, alternative therapy or natural treatment of perimenopause symptoms?

5. Are you willing to consult with other professionals on other possible treatments?

6. Will you review the pros and cons of hormone replacement therapy, including the pros and cons of synthetic and natural forms of estrogen?

7. What are your fees?

8. (If the doctor is part of a managed health care plan) How difficult is it to be referred to a specialist?

9. What is the procedure for after-hours calls?

10. With which hospital are you affiliated?

Of course, you should add any specific questions of your own you may have as well. After you've met with the prospective doctor, it's time to review the meeting and think about how the staff at this doctor's office made you feel and whether you would be comfortable returning for your regular care.

Ten Things to Think About After Your Visit

1. Was the doctor knowledgeable about menopause? (A gynecologist whose emphasis is in childbirth may not be as helpful or well informed in the areas of menopause and aging.)

2. How much time did the doctor spend with you?

3. Was there enough time to adequately explain your lifestyle issues and your family history?

4. Was the doctor readily available? Having to wait a month or more for an appointment may be too long. At the same time, having to wait in the waiting room may not be the doctor's fault—emergencies can happen. If you had an emergency, you would want the doctor to put aside his or her regular patients to see you.

5. Could you talk with the doctor openly, as an equal? Did the doctor call you by your first name but expect you to call him or her "Dr. Smith"?

6. How did the doctor respond to your questions?

7. Did it seem as if he or she would get upset if you questioned advice or information?

8. Did the doctor explain things in a way you can understand?

9. Is the doctor in a group or solo practice? Do you feel comfortable about the procedure for handling after-hours calls?

10. If the doctor can't speak to you when you call with a question, is there another trained person who can take the call (such as a physician's assistant or a nurse)?

Your relationship with your doctor is an important one. You should feel as comfortable and trusting with this person as you do with your lawyer or banker. If you feel uncomfortable for any reason, don't hesitate to discuss your feelings with the doctor or to seek another physician.

What's Next?

In the next chapter you'll learn about some treatments for perimenopausal symptoms that are different from the usual hormone replacement therapy. These treatments, referred to as "alternative treatments," can sometimes be a real help in combating symptoms without unpleasant or long-term side effects.

5 Alternative Treatment

As more than 40 million American women move into the perimenopause and menopause phases of their lives, many begin to grapple with the arguments for and against hormone replacement therapy. In fact, not all women need estrogen, and some women can't take it. Many doctors don't want to give hormones to women who are still having their periods, however erratically. Indeed, only a third of menopausal women in the United States try hormone replacement, and of those who do, eventually half of them drop the therapy. Some are worried about breast cancer, some can't tolerate the side effects, some are offended by their doctor's attempt to medicate what they consider to be a natural occurrence.

Instead, herbal teas and tablets for the midlife woman have started appearing not just in natural food stores, but in grocery store chains and pharmacies. More women are turning to alternative therapies, including homeopathy, naturopathy, acupuncture, massage, biofeedback, meditation, yoga, and herbal medicine, and these practices are starting to appear at women's health clinics across the country.

What's important is to look at alternative therapy as an individualized choice. Just as not all women can take hormones, not all women can just take herbs. A woman whose mother had osteoporosis, who has smoked all her life, and who is small boned and thin is at risk for significant bone loss herself. These days, her caregiver may be far more willing to choose therapies based not on whether it's traditional or alternative, but on what has the best chance of protecting this particular patient.

It's quite possible to have an occasional period yet still be wracked with hot flashes, headaches, moodiness, and many other perimenopausal symptoms. You're not menopausal—but you still have plenty of symptoms. Fortunately, there are alternative choices you can try that still carry the hope of easing your symptoms.

But perimenopausal women aren't the only ones interested in alternative methods of controlling symptoms. Menopausal women, women with a personal or family history of breast or uterine cancer, or women with active liver disease or active thrombophlebitis may prefer to choose an alternative treatment over HRT. Other women simply don't like the idea of taking hormones. Still others don't like to treat menopause as though it were a deficiency disease.

In Chapter 2 we discussed some of the lifestyle changes you can make to deal with a variety of perimenopausal-related symptoms. In this chapter we're going to explore some alternative remedies to these symptoms. These include vegetable estrogens, herbs, vitamins, and some nontraditional techniques such as homeopathy, acupressure, and acupuncture.

Plant-Derived Estrogens (phytoestrogens)

One alternative treatment that has been snagging plenty of media attention lately is the use of plant-derived hormones, also known as *phytoestrogens*. Calling phytoestrogens "close to a wonder drug" in her recent book, *Dr. Susan Love's Hormone Book*, Dr. Love—a controversial critic of HRT—has herself now entered perimenopause. To cope, she reports, she packs in the phytoestrogen-rich food (such as soybeans and flaxseed), doses herself with black cohosh (an herbal source of phytoestrogens), and exercises daily.

What concerns some critics of natural hormones and other alternative remedies is that many women think that "natural" means "harmless." That's not necessarily so. For example, in large doses, according to anecdotal reports, phytoestrogens can promote the abnormal growth of cells in the uterine lining. Unopposed estrogen of *any* type can lead to endometrial cancer, which is why women on conventional estrogen replacement therapy usually take progestin along with their estrogen (Premarin). Keep in mind that almost *any* substance—even table salt—can be toxic if taken in large doses.

There are three classes of phytoestrogens: isoflavones, lignans, and coumestans. Most plants contain phytoestrogens to some degree, but those that are most like human estrogen are the isoflavone-containing legumes such as soy products, lentils, and kidney or lima beans. Lignans are found in bread and cereal grains, fruits, and vegetables. Coumestans are found in alfalfa, seed sprouts, and fodder crops.

The major isoflavones are genistein, diadzein, and equol; primary lignans are enterolactone and enterodiol.

By binding to human estrogen receptors, they supplement the effects of estrogen when levels are low, and they interfere with the human estrogen (estradiol) when levels are high. This ability to adapt is why they appeal to perimenopausal women, whose hormones can fluctuate wildly prior to menopause.

Soy Products

Proponents of plant estrogens argue that some phytoestrogens appear to act as antigrowth factors in the uterus and breast. The results of smaller preliminary trials suggest that the estrogenic compounds that soy contains (genistein and diadzein) can relieve the severity of hot flashes and lower cholesterol. But no one yet has proven that soy can provide all the benefits of Premarin without its negative effects.

It is true that people in other countries who eat food high in phytoestrogens—especially soy products—experience a lower incidence of diseases such as cardiovascular disease, breast cancer, and prostate cancer. In fact, although up to 80 percent of perimenopausal U.S. women complain of hot flashes, night sweats, and vaginal dryness, only 15 percent of Japanese women have similar complaints. And women in Indonesia, India, and Taiwan likewise have much lower rates of heart disease, breast cancer, and hip fractures. When all other things are equal, the soy-based diet appears to make the difference—and soy is very high in phytoestrogens.

Blood levels of phytoestrogens are 10 to 40 times higher in Japanese women than in American women, and Japanese women experience hot flashes only one sixth as often. There isn't even a phrase in Japanese for "hot flash."

Studies have shown that soy consumption has reduced total cholesterol, "bad" cholesterol, and triglycerides without affecting "good" cholesterol. Experts suspect that soy may also protect against plaque in blood vessels and that it may (like estrogen) increase the flexibility of blood vessels.

Scientists have also tried studying how soy may be related to lower levels of breast cancer. For example, genistein, which functions a bit like tamoxifen and other "anti-estrogens," seems to be able to connect to the estrogen receptors on a breast cancer cell, effectively blocking estrogen's passage into the cell, denying tumor cells a powerful growth factor. A number of studies are now going on that would determine whether diets containing soy or genistein prevent breast cancer, but results will not be available for several years. Experts also discovered that women on a soy diet appeared to have a significant increase in bone density (limited to the spine), perhaps because the genistein spurred bone formation.

However, the study of phytoestrogens is so new that there aren't very many recommendations on how much a woman could consume. In one study at Bowman-Gray medical school in North Carolina, women were able to ease their symptoms by drinking a soy beverage with 20 mg of isoflavones. You could mimic that amount by eating a large amount of fruits, vegetables, and whole grains, together with four ounces of tofu (smooth-textured bean curd sold in cakes) four times a week.

You can find many different varieties of soy at natural food stores, which stock soy cheeses, soy milk, tofu, soy tempeh (made from whole soybeans and sold in a cake), soy powders and flours, and so on. Still, it's not easy to get as much tofu in your diet as you would if you ate like the Japanese. It's important to eat tofu not just once in a while but every day, to enjoy the protective benefits of the phytoestrogens.

Still, the data on soy is new. No one knows how soy interacts with estrogen supplements in birth control pills or in hormone replacement. And the isoflavone content of soy differs depending on the variety of bean and how it is used in processed food. In general, however, soy sauce and soy oils are low in isoflavones, whereas roasted soy nuts, tempeh, and tofu are high (about 40 mg per ½ c).

When you do start adding more soy products to your diet, add them slowly. If you get too much soy all at once, you may suffer from gas. Try to mimic the diet of the average Japanese woman—between 30 to 50 mgs of isoflavones per day—because the effects of eating larger amounts are unknown. (However, many Asians routinely consume up to 100 mg of isoflavones a day without apparent problems.)

When adding some of these soy products to your diet, don't forget that some products are very high in calories and sodium. And if you're wondering whether it's better to get your isoflavones in food or in capsules, experts suggest that just as betacarotene may not work if taken alone as a supplement, isoflavones may not either. It's also possible to overdose on isoflavone capsules. It's probably better, therefore, to eat soy products rather than take capsules.

POOR CHOICES FOR ISOFLAVONES

The following soy foods are *not* good sources of isoflavones:

- soy sauce

- soybean oil

- miso (contains only minute amounts of isoflavones)

- soy foods made from soy protein concentrate (such as many veggie burgers)

- "combination" food with soy and other ingredients (soy cheese, soy hot dogs, soy bacon, tofu yogurt, and canned meal-replacement drinks)

PHYTOESTROGEN-RICH FOODS

apples	hops	peppers (green)
asparagus	legumes	pomegranates
barley	licorice	rice bran
beans	linseed	rye
carrots	oat bran	seaweed (dried)
cereal	oats	soy products
cherries	olive oil	squash
corn	onions	stone fruits
fennel	pears	sunflower seeds
garlic	peas	wheat germ

ISOFLAVONE LEVELS

Food	Serving	Isoflavones
soy nuts (roasted)	¼ c	60
tempeh	½ c	35
tofu (low fat)	½ c	35
tofu (regular)	½ c	35
soy milk (regular)	1 c	30
soy milk (low fat)	1 c	25
soy butter (roasted)	2 tbsp	17

Bioflavonoids

Bioflavonoids have a mild estrogen effect and are used to treat vaginal dryness, bladder problems, water retention, and hot flashes. Highest concentration is found in the inner peel of citrus fruits, but they also occur in a wide variety of other sources. They are often taken with vitamin C.

Herbal Remedies

Women around the world have been using herbal remedies to relieve perimenopausal symptoms for centuries. They are not always the first choice of traditional physicians, in part because many herbs haven't been tested in strict, controlled studies. One of the main reasons why they haven't been tested is that there are no financial incentives to do so.

The FDA requires that any herb marketed as a medicine must meet the same stringent testing standards as a drug. It's hard to interest manufacturers in taking the time and expense to test and introduce herbs as medicine because they wouldn't be able to sell the herb for a high price if it were effective. After all, anyone can grow her own herbs in the backyard. Because a plant can't be patented, U.S. pharmaceutical companies sometimes choose to transform the active ingredient of an herb into a drug and patent that.

This is why most herbs are sold as food supplements, not medicines—which tends to give the impression that they aren't very effective. What this means is that some Americans dismiss the healing properties of herbs because they assume they are weak and ineffective, whereas others misuse or overdose on herbs because they assume they are weak and therefore harmless.

In Europe (especially Germany) herbs sold as medicine are strictly regulated, widely prescribed by physicians, dispensed only by licensed pharmacists, and covered by insurance when prescribed by a doctor.

In the United States, however, the lack of regulations on herbal products means there is a wide variety in quality. Because herbal products aren't regulated, contamination or accidental overdose is possible. When buying herbs, purchase them from a recognized company or through a qualified herbal practitioner. You can grow them yourself, but it can be more difficult to know precisely the amount and strength of the active ingredient.

In general, most herbs are safe, according to the American Association of Poison Control Centers, with no substantial evidence that herbal products are a major source of toxic reactions. Of course this doesn't mean that you can take as much of an herb as you want with perfect confidence. "The dose makes the poison," as old herbalists warn, which means that anything taken in excessive amounts can be harmful. You should learn all you can about herbs, and work with a qualified practitioner—an herbalist, a traditional Chinese doctor, or a naturopathic physician—to make sure what you're taking is both safe and effective. You should also be sure to let your primary care doctor know what you're taking.

If you are already taking any medications or you have any kind of health condition, you should discuss your interest in herbs with your doctor before taking anything. If you are pregnant, you should avoid these herbs because of unknown effects on a developing fetus. Likewise, be aware that as a natural substance, herbs have varying amounts of the effective component depending on soil and weather conditions. For these reasons it may be better to buy from a reputable dealer than to try to grow your own.

Many of the herbs used to treat perimenopausal symptoms are widely prescribed by herbalists and naturopathic physicians. Many contain some of the same plant hormones (phytoestrogens) as does tofu, although in much lower concentrations. They can raise a low level of estrogen while lowering a high level; for this reason they are known as "balancers."

Using herbs to treat perimenopausal symptoms does have some drawbacks, however. Many have particular side effects, although they will probably be milder than a side effect from drugs. Any herb also can trigger an allergic reaction in susceptible individuals. For this reason you should begin with one herb at a time and wait a bit before adding a second herb.

Most of these herbs can be found in health food stores, Asian specialty grocery stores, herb stores, or farmers' markets. You should take them in moderation, and if you experience any side effects, such as nausea, dizziness, stomach pains, diarrhea, headache, or blurred vision, after taking any of these herbs, stop taking them immediately.

The following list of herbs includes those that are most often prescribed by herbalists. This section discusses these herbs in general; later in the chapter, the "symptom-by-symptom" list explains dosages of these herbs needed to treat specific symptoms.

Black Cohosh

This herbal root (*Cimicifuga racemosa*), a member of the buttercup family, was the traditional favorite of Native American women suffering with menstrual problems, which is where one of its nicknames—squawroot—

originated. Also known as black snakeroot or bugbane, it supplies the building blocks for the steroid hormones such as estrogen, progesterone, and testosterone and is believed to have estrogenlike effects in the body, binding to estrogen receptors in the uterus.

It has been well studied in Germany, where it is contained in several prescription medications used for menopause complaints (especially hot flashes). In fact, in one German study women who took the capsule version of black cohosh (Remifemin) got as much relief from their symptoms as the women who took Premarin, and both groups of women fared better than those who took a placebo. Other experiments have shown that the herb has substances that can bind to estrogen receptors in animals. Black cohosh was an official drug in the *U.S. Pharmacopoeia* from 1820 to 1926.

Possible side effects (more often found in preparations from the dried or powdered root in capsules) include a worsening of heavy menstrual bleeding, headache, dizziness, visual disturbance, and nausea. You should not use black cohosh if you think you might be pregnant. You should not take black cohosh for more than six months because there is no information on long-term safety. Because of its estrogenlike effects, it is not a good choice for any woman who has breast cancer.

Blackberry Root

Taken in moderation, blackberry root can alleviate some perimenopausal symptoms.

Blackcurrant

Many women believe that blackcurrant oil can reduce the breast tenderness that can accompany perimenopause at certain times of the month. Although herbalists make use of the berries, seeds, leaves, and oil, today the oil is generally used for its rich source of essential fatty acids. There have been no reports of toxic effects.

Chasteberry or Chaste Tree (Vitex)

Many women swear by chasteberry as an herb, well known to ancient herbalists, that helps against hot flashes. "If blood flows from the womb," wrote Hippocrates, "let the woman drink dark wine in which the leaves of the Vitex have been steeped." This point of view was echoed by Pliny and Homer. It is believed to help balance and raise progesterone and estrogen levels, and can be used to help control menstrual bleeding. It may also help shrink fibroids. Several German studies have shown that it can be effective in alleviating some of the symptoms of PMS (which are very similar to perimenopausal symptoms). Herbalists note that you may have to take the herb for several weeks or months before you notice an improvement. You should generally take between 30 and 40 mg.

Although this drug doesn't usually cause side effects, you should tell your doctor if you plan to try this herb.

Dong Quai

A popular Asian choice for problems of the reproductive system, this herb (*Angelica sinensis*) is said to have an estrogenlike effect on the body and is used to even out high and low levels of estrogen in the body. It has extremely active phytoestrogens, and it may have some beneficial effects on your heart because it's a type of blood thinner. In one study of an herbal formula that includes dong quai (*dang gui shao yao san*), its ability to suppress estradiol secretion in rats suggests that it may be safe for women with breast cancer.

However, dong quai is always used in concert with a host of other herbs, so if you want to try it for perimenopausal symptoms, find a skilled herbalist to prescribe the right combination. Herbalists do recommend dong quai for the quick relief of hot flashes.

Dong quai can sensitize your skin to the sun. You should avoid this herb if you have heavy menstrual bleeding, take blood-thinning drugs, have fibroids or diarrhea, or feel bloated.

Evening Primrose Oil

Taken in moderation, primrose oil (made from the seeds of the primrose plant) can alleviate some perimenopause symptoms. More than 120 studies in 15 countries have reported on the potential use of the oil, which is high in the essential fatty acid gammalinolenic acid (GLA). One study found that supplementing the diet with evening primrose oil helped to relieve mood swings, irritability, and breast tenderness. However, at least one study found effects of the oil to be insignificant.

Some women who take evening primrose may experience stomach discomfort, nausea, or headache.

Fennel Seeds

Another herb with a mild estrogenlike effect on the body, fennel seeds have been used traditionally to trigger milk flow in nursing mothers. Some women also say it helps relieve hot flashes. Make a tea with a cup of boiling water over 1 or 2 teaspoons of crushed seeds and steep ten minutes. Drink up to three times a day.

Flaxseed

The seeds and oil of this herb (*Linum usitatissimum*) contain prostaglandins that can prevent excessive menstrual bleeding, but taking too much can lead to cramping. Used in the Middle East for the last seven thousand years, flaxseed is a good source of essential fatty acids. Rich in GLA, it is recommended for many of the symptoms of PMS and perimenopause, including breast tenderness. Also known as linseed oil, it must be fresh, and you should buy it in small amounts and keep it refrigerated. Tell your doctor if you use this herb.

Gingko Biloba

Herbalists believe this Chinese herb can boost memory, and in at least one study it did appear to have some benefit on people suffering with age-related memory problems. Also known as the maidenhair tree, gingko is one of the oldest tree species on earth and is widely cultivated in the United States. In Chinese medicine it has been used for its beneficial effects on the brain since 2800 B.C.

In more than fifty double-blind studies, scientists found gingko helped reduce vascular insufficiency and age-related decrease in brain function. This herb may help improve the memory problems experienced by many perimenopausal women; others use the herb together with hawthorn to improve memory. Gingko is nontoxic.

Ginseng

A popular tonic for hot flashes, ginseng contains hormonelike compounds that mimic estrogen. Available in tinctures, teas, and tonics, ginseng is an ancient Korean root that has been used by Asians for seven thousand years to enhance vitality. It has been shown to prevent the thinning of the vagina seen in perimenopause, and may help relieve fatigue that often accompanies the onset of these symptoms.

However, doctors are often reluctant to prescribe ginseng for the alleviation of perimenopausal symptoms because it is rather like taking estrogen replacement without any idea of exactly how much estrogen you're getting.

Getting what you pay for with ginseng can be a problem; most ginseng products contain only a trace of the active ingredient (ginsenoside), and some don't contain any. When you buy it, check out the amount of ginsenoside the product contains. Ginseng is available in a number of forms, including:

- Asian ginseng (*Panax schinseng*)

- American ginseng (*Panax quinquefolius*)

- tienchi ginseng (*Panax pseudoginseng*)

- Siberian ginseng (*Eleutherococcus senticosus*)

The American variety is recommended by herbalist Susun Weed, author of *The Menopausal Years: The Wise Woman Way*. Dosages vary according to the amount of active ingredient and your weight; the easiest way to figure out what dose you're getting is to buy ginseng in capsules. Some herbalists recommend 500 mg twice a day if you weigh less than 130 lb, three times a day for those up to 160 lb, and four times daily for those over 160 lb; however, it is best to ask your doctor about dosage. When in doubt, take ginseng only in moderation and not for long.

Ginseng works best on an empty stomach; experts recommend that you don't eat fruit for two hours after taking ginseng, and that you take it separately from any other vitamin supplement, especially vitamin C (it isn't well absorbed with acid). However, its effects can be boosted if you take it with vitamin E or flaxseed oil.

Note: Ginseng is a stimulant. Overdoses can lead to insomnia and anxiety, and can cause an unpleasant jittery, overstimulated feeling. It can also cause postmenopausal bleeding—stop using this herb if this happens to you.

Other side effects include high blood pressure, breast tenderness, diarrhea, insomnia, nervousness, and skin problems, and it can worsen a fever. *This herb should not be used by anyone with:*

- asthma

- blood-clotting problems

- cardiac arrhythmia

- emphysema

- high blood pressure

- fever

- diabetes

Hawthorn

This popular "heart herb" also may improve memory and thinking, conditions that are often described as "fuzzy" by perimenopausal women. Also known as May bush, the hawthorn is a thorn tree, with bright red berries, that grows 25 feet tall. Used since the Middle Ages as a heart tonic, hawthorn dilates blood vessels and improves circulation. It is sometimes used together with *gingko biloba* to diminish menopausal memory loss.

Lady's Mantle

A popular German treatment for excessive menstrual bleeding, lady's mantle is taken a couple of weeks before your period. Tell your doctor before you take this herb.

Motherwort

Herbalists use the bitter-tasting *Leonurus cardiaca* to ease night sweats and hot flashes. Because it appears to have slight estrogenic effects, it's best to avoid motherwort if you have breast cancer. Women who have heavy bleeding should not use this plant because it may increase bleeding. You can take 15 to 25 drops of tincture of the fresh flowering plant up to six times a day.

Oatstraw

This popular herb is believed by many herbalists to help ease nerves, and therefore to be useful for controlling mood swings in perimenopausal women.

Red Clover

This herb is reported to ease hot flashes because it acts like estrogen in the body.

Sage

A plant that contains both bioflavonoids and phytoesterols, sage acts like a weak estrogen and has been used for mood swings, headaches, and night sweats, among other things. Herbalists suggest that women with breast cancer should not take this herb.

In addition to its use as a condiment, you can make sage tea with one or two spoonfuls of dried leaf infusion one to eight times a day, or 15 to 40 drops of fresh leaf tincture up to three times a day. Don't take more than this dose, or you risk harming your kidneys and liver.

Valerian

The *Valeriana officinalis* is a powerful sedative plant that can become habit forming. If taken, it should be taken before bedtime to aid sleep.

Wild Mexican Yam Root

The wild Mexican yam (also known as Devil's bones or colic root) was used by the Native Americans for birth control. Today, extracts from wild Mexican yam are available in creams, pills, and suppositories. The herb's root contains a natural form of DHEA (dehydroepiandrosterone) similar to progesterone that many women have been enthusiastically recommending for the treatment of vaginal dryness, hot flashes, and a host of other peri-menopausal symptoms. Most commonly prescribed synthetic hormones are made from the diosgenin found in the wild yam. However, there is no evidence that your body can transform diosgenin into progesterone, although the root does have some effects in balancing your cycle. It is a popular herb used for hundreds of years by Native Americans to ease labor pains.

The cream should be applied twice a day during the second half of your menstrual cycle if you are still having periods. Because some wild yam creams also contain progesterone as an additional ingredient, you must read the label to make sure you know what you are getting.

Because many women mistakenly assume that "natural" means "harmless," it is important to remember that any substance taken in too high a dose can be toxic. Be very cautious about using too much of this product or too often; it's very hard to control the dosage of a skin cream, and too much natural progesterone—just like its synthetic cousin—can cause fluid buildup, irritability, and weight gain.

Acupuncture

As discussed in Chapter 4, the ancient Asian art of acupuncture is usually painless and has been used for many perimenopausal symptoms, including insomnia, hot flashes, and irregular periods. There are a number of American schools of acupuncture and Chinese medicine, and a national Council of Acupuncturist Schools and Colleges that regulates the training and education of practitioners. The National Commission for the Certi-fication of Acupuncturists helps ensure competence.

Acupressure and Massage

Therapeutic massage involving acupressure can bring relief from a wide range of perimenopause symptoms. Acupressure involves placing finger pressure at the same meridian points on the body that are used in acupuncture.

There are more than eighty different types of massage, including foot reflexology, shiatsu massage, and Swedish massage. They are all based on the idea that boosting the circulation of blood and lymph benefits health. Massage therapists also believe that because most chronic illnesses are related to stress, relieving stress will help the chronic condition. During the massage, your tight muscles relax and the pain that comes with chronic tension dissolves. Massage can ease the effects of stress by helping to:

- lower heart rate and blood pressure
- improve circulation
- raise skin temperature
- heighten sense of well-being
- reduce anxiety level

You can find a good certified or well-trained massage therapist by contacting the American Massage Therapy Association.

Biofeedback

Some women have been able to control their hot flashes by using biofeedback, a painless technique in which you are attached to a machine that can help you train your mind to take control of your body's mechanisms.

The machine provides you with tones or meter readings of the body mechanism you're trying to control, such as skin temperature, heart rate, or muscle tension. As you learn to relax, you can actually control the speed of your beating heart or the temperature of the skin on your hands.

Homeopathy

Homeopathic physicians use dilute solutions of naturally occurring substances that if given in full strength would provoke the same symptoms the patient is being treated for—the doctrine that "like cures like," or the law of similars. The concept is based on the idea of the existence of vital energy, roughly akin to the traditional Chinese belief of *chi*. This means that when you are in balance, you're healthy, but when this harmony is destroyed, your symptoms are your body's way of trying to regain its *chi*. For this reason you should not try to suppress symptoms, according to homeopaths.

Western medicine tries to cure disease by destroying the cause of the disease; eastern medicine tries to strengthen and balance the body to fight the disease on its own. A homeopathic approach tries to provoke the body to strengthen itself so the body can heal itself. Homeopathic physicians treat many of the perimenopausal symptoms.

Critics say that homeopathic remedies are too dilute to have any effects at all, and that any positive results are simply the result of the placebo effect. Although there have been no studies of homeopathic treatments of menopause symptoms, a few studies have suggested that the treatments appear to have some mild benefits. Still, scientists have no real proof why, or how, homeopathy works.

Homeopathic practitioners are not licensed in homeopathy although most experts are licensed providers in other health care specialties, including chiropractors, naturopaths, acupuncturists, nurses, nurse practitioners, physician's assistants, M.D.s, pharmacists, or dentists. You do need to find a homeopathic practitioner with whom to work because treatment is highly individualized; you must match treatment to your symptoms. This is why buying a homeopathic remedy at a store without working with an expert may not be the best way to treat your symptoms.

Naturopathy

This tradition combines a variety of natural treatments so that the body can heal itself. The naturopathic physician must treat the whole patient, using a variety of healing practices including diet, homeopathy, acupuncture, herbal medicine, exercise, spinal and soft-tissue manipulation, physical therapy, counseling, and medication.

Because the naturopathic philosophy treats the whole person, it can be a good choice for perimenopausal women looking for symptom relief. Naturopathic physicians are licensed in 13 states in the United States and in Canada. You can obtain referrals from the American Association of Naturopathic Physicians.

Yoga

It may seem far-fetched, but many women find that yoga—the ancient practice developed in India five thousand years ago—can help with perimenopausal symptoms. Yoga focuses on uniting the mind, body, and spirit to create balance in your life and is considered to be a form of meditation.

Because yoga has been shown to balance the endocrine system, some experts believe it may affect hormone-related problems. Studies have found that yoga can reduce stress, improve mood, boost sluggish metabolism, and slow heart rate.

Specific yoga positions deal with particular problems, such as hot flashes, mood swings, vaginal and urinary problems, and other pains.

You can start yoga at any age. Before beginning, you should check with your doctor if you are overweight or have high blood pressure, arthritis, or a back injury. For women who have trouble finding time for exercise, fitting in a 15-minute session of stretching and breathing may have a powerful impact on your health.

Symptom-by-Symptom List of Alternative Treatment

Bleeding (excessive or erratic)

- acupuncture

- chasteberry or chaste tree: 20 drops of tincture once or twice per day; *or* 3 capsules of fresh powdered berries per day; *or* 1 cup of tea

- vitamin C

- lady's mantle: 5–10 drops of fresh plant tincture three times per day up to two weeks a month (before your period); it can help control bleeding once it starts, but it takes up to five days to become effective

- flaxseed: drink 1–3 tbsp oil in the morning, *or* grind seeds and eat on cereal

- wild yam root: 2–4 drops of tincture per day one to two weeks before your period; may help decrease bleeding (tell your doctor if you take this herb)

- herbs to avoid if you bleed heavily: black cohosh, dong quai, motherwort

Bloated Feeling

- Primrose oil may be effective in helping to treat your bloating and cramps.

- vitamin B_6

Breast Changes

Vitamin B_6 can offset the problem of tender breasts; it is considered a natural diuretic.

Depression

It's important to note the difference between symptom-related feelings of depression and emotional illness. Today experts don't believe that perimenopause and menopause cause depression. If you are feeling depressed, you need to talk to a mental health care expert about treatment for depression—not for perimenopause.

Facial Hair

There are many ways to remove facial hair, but electrolysis is the only permanent way to remove this hair. Temporary methods include tweezing, shaving, waxing, or using a depilatory.

Fatigue

- vitamin B_6: 50–100 mg per day

- vitamin E (together with vitamin B complex, potassium, magnesium, bioflavonoids): 800 mg per day

Headache

- Wild yam cream rubbed on the back of the neck may ease hormone-related migraines.

Hot Flashes

- Thousands of women report that vitamin E can ease hot flashes, although studies have not yet provided conclusive proof. Begin with 800 mg per day, and don't take more than 1,000 mg a day (see Chapter 8). *Because vitamin E can raise blood pressure, consult your doctor before taking it.*

- one vitamin B-50 complex tablet and 500 mg of vitamin C every day

- acupuncture, meditation, and biofeedback for relief from hot flashes (see earlier discussion)

- bee pollen: 500 mg, 3 tablets per day

- bioflavonoids: 250 mg, five or six times per day

- Chickweed tincture (25–40 drops) once or twice a day can reduce the severity and frequency of hot flashes.

- dandelion: 1,000–3,000 mg in capsule form daily; *or* 2–3 cups of tea daily; *or* 1–2 tsp of dandelion tincture three times per day

- dong quai: 10–40 drops of fresh root tincture up to three times per day, *or* 4–8 oz of dried root infusion *or* tea daily (see earlier cautions)

- elderflower (Sambucus species): 25–50 drops of fresh blossom tincture several times per day

- ginseng (see earlier discussion)

- herbs commonly used to alleviate hot flashes: anise, black or blue cohosh, chasteberry, fennel, wild yam root, licorice root, false unicorn, red clover, or sarsaparilla

- motherwort extract: 25–40 drops every four hours

- sage tea: several cups a day, using 1 tbsp of sage per cup of water

- soy products (such as tofu)

- viola: make an infusion from dried leaves, and drink at least 1 cup a day

- yoga (see earlier discussion)

Insomnia

- vitamin/mineral supplements—vitamins B (50–100 mg), C (500 mg), and E (800 mg); calcium (800–1200 mg) and copper (2–3 mg)

- herbal teas (especially chamomile, catnip, or mint)

- acupuncture/acupressure (see earlier discussion)

- motherwort

- valerian: 20–30 drops just before bedtime (but note that valerian can be habit forming)

Irritability/Mood Swings

- vitamin B complex: 50–100 mg, to relieve stress

- calcium: increasing intake to 1,300 mg a day may make you feel calmer

- relaxation techniques (see Chapter 8)
- vitamin E: 800 mg
- motherwort: 5–10 drops
- yoga (see earlier discussion)

Loss of Sexual Interest

- Many of the tips used to ease the pain of vaginal dryness can go a long way toward boosting your interest in sex.
- ginseng

Night Sweats

Ginseng is a popular remedy for night sweats in doses of 1,000 mg daily. Ginseng is also a stimulant; overdoses can lead to insomnia and anxiety.

Palpitations

Dong quai may help calm palpitations.

Thinking and Memory Problems

- vitamin B complex
- sage
- ginseng (sharpens mental abilities and memory): 5–40 drops of fresh root tincture three times per day, *or* 4–8 oz dried root infusion *or* tea daily
- *Gingko biloba*

Urinary Changes

- yoga (see earlier discussion)

- biofeedback (for stress incontinence)

- black cohosh: 1 cup of tea a day *or* 10–60 drops of tincture per day

Vaginal Dryness

- motherwort tincture: take for three to seven days to improve lubrication

- vitamin E (together with vitamin B complex, potassium, magnesium, bioflavonoids): 800 mg

- wild yam: 2–4 ml of tincture per day

- yoga

- ginseng

- vitamin E, according to some women

- primrose oil (available in capsule form)

What's Next?

If you find that alternative methods don't work for you, the next chapter provides a full discussion on the different methods of hormone replacement therapy (HRT). This controversial method involves taking progesterone and estrogen together to treat the symptoms of perimenopause. But there are many ways to manipulate the levels of these and other hormones to best suit your body and lifestyle. A list of pros and cons and common side effects of each method, along with the advice of your physician, can help you decide if HRT is a viable option.

6 Hormone Replacement Therapy

One of the most controversial aspects of health care in midlife is the issue of hormone replacement. As you approach menopause, you may experience a wide range of symptoms associated with falling levels of estrogen and progesterone: hot flashes, night sweats, dry vagina, incontinence, decreased interest in sex—together with an increased risk of osteoporosis and heart disease.

Hormone replacement therapy seeks to balance those levels by replacing what is lost. When estrogen alone is prescribed, it's called simply "estrogen replacement therapy," or ERT); the amount of estrogen that is replaced is only a fraction of the amount of estrogen the ovary used to produce on its own.

If you still have your uterus when you enter perimenopause, your doctor won't want to give you estrogen replacement alone; adding progesterone prevents any increase in the risk of uterine cancer from the "unopposed" estrogen supplements. When a woman takes progesterone (or the synthetic progestin) in addition to estrogen, that is known as hormone replacement therapy (HRT).

Most physicians don't recommend hormone replacement therapy until your periods have stopped for one year. If you are perimenopausal, chances are your ovaries are still producing estrogen. HRT would then provide far too much estrogen, causing a buildup in the lining of the uterus and possibly creating a precancerous condition. The decision about whether or not to undertake HRT is up to you and your doctor. This chapter explores the role of hormone replacement because it is likely that many women, at some point during their lives, will consider HRT.

Birth Control Pills as HRT

There is another choice for women who are still having their periods but whose symptoms won't go away just by making lifestyle changes in diet, exercise, and so on. For these women, low-dose birth control pills (popularly called "the Pill") can solve some of these problems.

As explained earlier, many doctors don't like to prescribe hormone replacement for women who are still getting their periods because they may still be producing some estrogen; adding more hormones could lead to a higher risk of endometrial cancer. After perimenopause, HRT is safer because women are no longer producing any estrogen at all.

However, oral contraceptives in low doses can produce regular, predictable cycles and can regulate the erratic release of estrogen. The Pill suppresses the body's production of estrogen and progesterone, replacing it with a predetermined dose of both. By reining in this burst of estrogen, the Pill can ease hot flashes, vaginal dryness, and insomnia. Taking birth control pills prevents fluctuating hormone levels; you would continue to get your monthly period. When an FSH test reveals that you have arrived at menopause, you would simply stop taking the Pill. (A side benefit: it can protect against unexpected pregnancy, which can occur during perimenopause.)

In fact, low-dose oral contraceptives have been approved by the FDA as a treatment for perimenopausal symptoms in women under age 55. However, the Pill is not prescribed as often as it might be because of concerns about a possible link between stroke in older women and oral contraceptives. Although an analysis of the effect of birth control pills on the risk of breast cancer found no increased risk among women aged 24 to 39, there was a risk for both younger and older women who took the Pill. Women aged 46 to 54 had double the risk of breast cancer; once they stopped the Pill, the additional risk disappeared after three years. Women who smoke, however, should consider another alternative, because the Pill increases the risk of heart attack and stroke in smokers.

Moreover, some women just don't get relief with the Pill, and others can't tolerate the side effects—bloating, moodiness, and weight gain.

How Estrogen Works in the Body

Each ovary produces estrogen, one of the female hormones responsible for the development of female sex characteristics at puberty. When you enter perimenopause, your levels of estrogen drop and the annoying symptoms of perimenopause begin. HRT seeks to boost those levels enough to suppress the symptoms while also providing protection against heart disease, breast cancer, and osteoporosis.

Many women in the early days of perimenopause don't have symptoms that are severe enough to be significant, but you may want to consider hormone replacement if your symptoms are severe. Almost every expert agrees that the choice of HRT must be made by a woman and her doctor after taking into consideration her own unique medical history and situation. There is no one right answer for everyone.

HRT: Yes or No?

One of the most controversial subjects in the field of menopause is the question about the value of hormone replacement therapy. Women have been interested in HRT ever since the late 1960s when large numbers of women embraced estrogen replacement as a sort of Fountain of Youth. But within ten years, early optimism evaporated when the *New England Journal of Medicine* published two studies showing a strong link between estrogen replacement therapy and uterine cancer.

By the early 1980s doctors realized that by combining estrogen with progestin, they could mimic a woman's functioning ovaries and avoid the danger of uterine cancer that arose when women took estrogen alone. Nevertheless, the legacy of that earlier link between estrogen and cancer was hard for women and doctors to forget. Fewer than 20 percent of eligible women today use hormone replacement therapy, although interest is growing as more women of the baby boom generation enter perimenopause.

Hormone replacement therapy is still controversial, however, and leading experts often come to opposite conclusions about benefits and risks of the treatment method. Most experts do agree that perimenopause and menopause are not diseases that need to be cured, but a natural life-stage transition that has become inappropriately burdened with negative symbolism.

Some doctors believe that all women (except those with certain cancers) should take hormones as they approach menopause because of the protection against heart disease, osteoporosis, and uterine cancer and the low risk of breast cancer. Critics of HRT say that the benefits of taking hormonal drugs to ease symptoms isn't worth the risk—however small—that you might develop breast cancer. They argue that menopause isn't a disease and that not *all* women should automatically be given hormones to "cure" what is actually a very natural process of aging.

The safety and wisdom of HRT, even for women already in menopause, are controversial. In recent years many studies on breast cancer and estrogen use have been conducted with conflicting results. Two 1995 studies that appeared in the *Journal of the American Medical Association* and the *New England Journal of Medicine* came to opposite conclusions about whether or not giving replacement estrogen to menopausal women increased the risk of breast cancer. After these studies were published, scientists at the National Institutes of Health advised women to consult their "medical caregiver for advice that is based on the individual's own personal health profile."

The Nurses Health Study by researchers at Brigham and Women's Hospital and Harvard Medical School concluded that short-term use of hormones carries little risk, whereas HRT used for more than five years among women 55 and over carries a 40 percent increase in risk of breast cancer.

If you do receive estrogen therapy, your physician will likely advise you to have regular breast exams, perform monthly self-exams, and have yearly mammograms after age 50.

Years ago, when a woman's life span was shorter, taking hormones didn't present such a problem. But because women today often survive into their mid-80s, taking replacement hormones and never going off them—as some doctors recommend—means taking hormones for a full third of their life. Doctors who recommend this say that menopause is a disease, and that hormone replacement is the cure.

Those experts who believe that menopause is a natural state with some temporary unpleasant symptoms recommend taking hormones for the few years when symptoms are difficult, gradually tapering off after menopause is complete. For those who see HRT as the answer to heart disease and osteoporosis, some experts prefer to prescribe HRT for women in their 60s who are at imminent risk of developing those diseases, rather than prescribing it for all healthy women in their 40s on the chance that a few of them might develop these problems. (It's worth noting that only one out of 25 women will get osteoporosis, for example.)

Pros and Cons of Hormone Replacement Therapy

1. Disease Risks and Benefits

Pro:

There are risks with HRT, and there are risks without it. If you don't have cancer in your family and your risk of dying from heart disease is high, then your low risk of cancer might be worth the protective benefit of avoiding heart disease. What is clear is that according to the 1991 study of 49,000 nurses published in the *New England Journal of Medicine*, the risk of dying of heart disease is far greater than the risk of dying of breast cancer for white women aged 50 to 94—these women were *eight times* more likely to die of heart disease than of breast cancer.

HRT may protect against heart disease, osteoporosis, Alzheimer's disease, and memory loss. It also can provide almost immediate relief from hot flashes, insomnia, fatigue, and low sex drive.

Con:

There is a real risk that HRT may be linked with cancer. Why take the risk to get rid of some unpleasant, yet transitory, symptoms? Is it sensible to swap the risk of a broken wrist for the risk of a diagnosis of breast cancer? Experts are concerned about the diseases that estrogen replacement might cause, including an increased risk of ovarian and uterine cancer in addition to breast cancer.

A few long-term studies have found that estrogen users—with or without the addition of progestin—face a greater risk of breast cancer than other women do. There may also be risks of lung and skin cancers, gallbladder problems, lupus and asthma, high blood pressure, liver disease, and blood-clotting problems.

2. Safety

Pro:

There are no studies that show that HRT can cause health problems when used for less than five years.

Con:

There has not been enough long-term testing to prove that HRT is a safe disease preventive when used for many years.

3. Is It "Natural" to Avoid Menopause?

Pro:

Maybe it's not "natural" to live this long, either. In the beginning of this century the average woman lived to be 50 years old; today the average age is 80. It doesn't make sense to use modern medicine to prolong a woman's life and then balk at improving the quality of that life. Taking hormones is replacing something that was lost, not introducing a totally new substance.

Con:

Hormone replacement therapy isn't natural. If women were meant to have hormones all their lives, they wouldn't go through menopause in the first place.

HRT Consensus

Most doctors agree that *short-term* use of estrogen for menopausal women with annoying symptoms of hot flashes or night sweats who don't have a history of breast cancer is a sensible choice. For perimenopausal women most experts would say that only if the woman is seriously troubled with symptoms should she consider HRT; for some of these women birth control pills might be a better solution, at least until the menstrual periods stop.

"I think it's important for women who choose estrogen therapy for relief of hot flashes or night sweats not to feel that this is a bad choice," writes HRT critic Susan Love, M.D., in *Dr. Susan Love's Hormone Book.* "No studies have found that short-term use of estrogen is dangerous and it can certainly improve your quality of life."

Is HRT Right for You?

As you've seen from the preceding discussion, hormone replacement therapy seems a bit like a two-edged sword. On the one hand, HRT can protect your bones and heart, but on the other hand, it might cause breast or uterine cancer. How do you decide whether HRT is right for you? By following the latest medical studies, finding a physician who will discuss the controversy in an open-minded way, and weighing the risk factors against your lifestyle and your own family history. After all that, you must be the one to make the final decision.

Experts suggest up to a third of women don't need hormone replacement therapy. Some perimenopausal women appear to be able to make their own estrogen, convert estrogen from other hormones, or use estrogen stored in fatty tissue. These are usually the women who don't have many symptoms. Perimenopausal women whose symptoms are severe, and who have no medical reason not to take hormones, may choose HRT.

Tara and Barbara are two women in their 40s who are suffering from significant perimenopausal symptoms. Tara's family medical background includes osteoporosis, heart disease, and uterine and colon cancer—but no incidence of breast cancer. As a result, Tara is thinking more seriously about how HRT could help her because it appears to protect against the very diseases that are common in her family, and she's not at risk for breast cancer, which has been linked to HRT.

On the other hand, Barbara's relatives had almost no problems from heart disease or osteoporosis—but almost every single one of her closest relatives did suffer with cancer: her grandmother, mother, and sister all had breast cancer, and her father and all four of his sisters died from cancer. For her the link between HRT and breast cancer—however tenuous—was disconcerting, especially because she did not appear to be at much risk for the diseases that HRT would protect against. The facts that her mother died of breast cancer and that her sister had breast cancer twice at an early age place her at very high risk for developing breast cancer even without the added risk of HRT.

If you do decide to take hormones, you should follow these tips to minimize the risks:

- Have an annual mammogram, breast exam, and pelvic exam.

- Tell your doctor at once if you have unusual vaginal bleeding or spotting (a sign of possible uterine cancer).

- If you have an intact uterus and you take estrogen without progestin, ask your doctor about an annual biopsy of the uterine lining.

GOOD CANDIDATES FOR HRT

HRT might be a good choice for you if you:

- need to prevent osteoporosis
- have had your ovaries removed
- need to prevent heart disease
- have several perimenopausal symptoms

POOR CANDIDATES FOR HRT

You would be a poor candidate for HRT if you:

- have ever been diagnosed with estrogen-positive breast cancer
- have had endometrial cancer
- have had gallbladder or liver disease
- have blood clots or phlebitis
- have a close relative (mother, sister, grandmother) who died of breast cancer

Note: Some women with liver or gallbladder disease or who have clotting problems may be able to go on HRT if they use the patch to bypass processing by the liver. Discuss the patch with your physician.

WHO SHOULD ABSOLUTELY AVOID HRT

You should definitely never go on hormone replacement therapy if you:

- have ever had breast cancer
- have two relatives who got breast cancer before age 40

Women at Slight Risk If Taking HRT

You may not want to take HRT if you have a history of the following conditions. You need to discuss HRT with your doctor if you have:

- blood clots or stroke (history of)
- deep vein thrombosis
- diabetes
- endometriosis
- fibroids (see note)
- gallstones, kidney disease, or liver disease (only if you are using the patch)
- high blood pressure
- obesity
- migraines
- pulmonary blockage
- sickle-cell anemia
- varicose veins

Note: In the past doctors counseled against HRT for women with benign fibroids in breast or uterus, but today's low-dosage estrogen in replacement therapy means you may be able to use HRT. Discuss your situation with your doctor.

Side Effects of HRT

Taking hormones to replace the ones you have lost can almost immediately eliminate hot flashes, vaginal dryness, urinary incontinence, insomnia, moodiness, heavy irregular periods, and memory and concentration problems. It sounds like a wonder drug, and some women do think of it as a sort of "youth pill."

Unfortunately, there are side effects that can include bloating, break-through bleeding, headaches, vaginal discharge, fluid retention, swollen breasts, and nausea. Up to 20 percent of women who try hormone replacement stop within nine months because of these side effects. Of course, the dosage and the method of HRT can influence the side effect profile. If your therapy includes progesterone (the hormone that induces your periods) in addition to estrogen, your side effects may include fluid retention, breast tenderness, moodiness, and headaches.

About one in four women say they gain weight on estrogen replacement, and many insist the hormone makes them hungrier. However, estrogen itself will not increase your weight.

Some women on estrogen replacement find that if they spend much time in the sun, patches of colored pigment appear on their faces. For this reason and because of the risk of skin cancer (whether or not you're taking hormones), it's a good idea to use a sunblock of at least SPF 15 in strength, and cover up with sunglasses and hat.

Finally, a recent study found that a mere two glasses of wine could more than double the amount of estrogen in the blood of women on HRT who have passed through menopause. Tell your doctor about your drinking habits if you are thinking about taking estrogen.

Most women may discover that it can be hard to find just the right dosage of hormones, and find themselves returning again and again to their doctor's office. It appears as if this tinkering is critical to getting the most out of your hormone replacement therapy because it's possible to adjust not just the dose, but the method of administration—pill, patch, injection, and so on. The goal is to find the lowest possible dose that will control your symptoms and protect you from heart disease and osteoporosis. Even in the best of cases most women should count on three to five return visits to get the adjustment just right.

How Much Is Too Much?

Women who had unpleasant symptoms when taking birth control pills years ago may assume that they aren't good candidates for HRT, but it's important to realize that the amount of estrogen needed to suppress ovulation is much higher than the amount required to ease perimenopause symptoms. This is why women who couldn't take the Pill because of the risk of blood clots may be able to have HRT.

When your ovaries were producing estradiol before perimenopause, your blood levels usually fluctuated between 40 pg/ml (picograms per milliliter) and 400 pg/ml during your cycle. A blood level of 50 to 65 pg/ml is usually enough to ease symptoms and protect your heart and bones.

If all you want is to get some relief from your hot flashes during your menopause years, you can take HRT for a few years and then gradually wean yourself off the hormones. If you're troubled with vaginal dryness or atrophy, you may need a longer treatment regimen, but still you should not need treatment for more than about four years.

HRT Regimens

There are just about as many ways to take hormones as there are symptoms of perimenopause. These include the following forms.

Oral Hormone Pill

Pills are portable, neat, and easy to take, and it's easy to manipulate dosage of a pill. However, when you take hormones by mouth, the pills are processed by the liver—which can boost the liver's production of clotting factors. This puts you at risk for blood clots, although the risk is fairly low unless you have a history of thrombosis or blood clots. Placing a pill under your tongue may help ease nausea. If you get nauseated from the pill, try taking it at bedtime.

Vaginal Hormone Pill

If you're having trouble tolerating estrogen in pill form or you are allergic to the skin patch, you can try inserting the estrogen pill (Estrace) into your vagina. It's easier to control the dosage this way than with a cream, and your body will still absorb enough medication to protect your heart and bones.

Skin Patch

One of the most popular new ways to administer hormones these days is with the skin patch (or transdermal patch), which provides a constant supply of estrogen while avoiding the liver. The transparent patch, which is about the size of a silver dollar, must be changed every three to four days. You can wear it on your abdomen or buttocks, where it delivers estrogen through the skin in a slow, even dose—just as your ovaries would do if they were still functioning at peak efficiency.

Although the patch is available in the United States in 0.05-mg and 0.1-mg doses, a lower dose of 0.025-mg, available in Europe, is not sold here. If you want to start out with an initially lower dose (to ease initial side effects), try placing a Band-Aid under the 0.05-mg patch to reduce the amount of estradiol that enters your bloodstream.

The patch is handy—you don't have to worry about taking a pill—and it is helpful for women with liver diseases. It's also easy to change dosages.

Unfortunately, some women are allergic to the adhesive on the patch. And although you can swim and bathe with the patch on, it may not stay on for long-term tub soaks. If you like to go long-distance swimming or use a hot tub, you can remove the patch and reapply it when the skin is dry. If you live in a hot, humid climate, you may have trouble keeping the patch on your skin; paper tape can help hold the patch in place in this case.

If the patch bothers your skin, remove it and try putting it on a new spot. However, if you experience a continued sensitivity to the adhesive, you may need to find another form of HRT.

If you notice that your symptoms continue even if you are using the higher-dose patch, ask your doctor to check your estradiol blood levels. Some women have problems absorbing the estradiol from the patch.

Vaginal Cream

If you suffer from vaginal dryness, you may want to consider a hormone cream that is inserted into the vagina. This form of HRT is used mostly for problems of the vaginal area or the urinary tract. If you opt for this method, have patience—it can take a long time to heal a dry, atrophied vagina. Women with this problem who are taking other forms of hormones may want to add vaginal cream to relubricate the vagina.

Although some of the hormones are absorbed into the bloodstream from the vagina, the levels aren't high enough to protect you against heart disease and osteoporosis. Dosage is usually a quarter of an applicator each day for four weeks, followed by an occasional dose every couple of days per week afterward. After a few months, the oral or patch forms of estrogen should be enough to keep the vagina lubricated.

Women like the speed of response when using the cream, but it can be difficult to apply and can cause unpleasant breast tenderness. Moreover, you shouldn't use the cream right before sex (your partner could absorb the cream through the penis and end up with side effects, such as enlarged breasts).

Injection

If you hate taking pills, have trouble remembering to change a patch, and find creams messy, you may want to consider once-a-month estradiol injections. The problem with these (besides the shot itself, which some women find unpleasant) is that you can't adjust the dosage once you've gotten the shot, even if you develop side effects.

Vaginal Ring

The FDA approved the progesterone ring Estring in April 1996. Once inserted into the top of the vagina, it gradually releases the hormone for up to three months. It can be easily removed if there is a problem, and it provides constant levels as long as it is in place.

Not Yet Approved

Crystalline 17b-estradiol pellets have not yet been approved by the FDA, but are used in Europe. The pellets can be surgically implanted under the skin so the estrogen is absorbed directly into the blood, bypassing the liver. The pellets can remain in place for up to six months.

The good news about this method is that you don't need to think about your hormones for six months. The bad news is that the pellets can be hard to remove if you are having side effects or other problems. Some women also have developed a tolerance to the high levels of estradiol in the pellets, and need more frequent insertion or higher doses.

HRT Dosage Regimens

There is a variety of ways to schedule your HRT, and the method you choose may depend in large part on whether or not you want to deal with a regular period. Women who take estrogen alone won't have a period, but adding progestin will bring on bleeding if you take it cyclically (not continuously).

Continuous Estrogen

If your uterus has been removed, you can take estrogen each day (usually as a skin patch or in a pill) because you are at no risk of getting uterine cancer. However, recent research suggests that progestin may also protect you from breast cancer in addition to uterine cancer. If this turns out to be the case, more women now taking estrogen alone may want to try the combination.

Cyclic Estrogen

Once a popular method of taking estrogen alone, it's not used often today because this method can trigger perimenopausal symptoms in the days when you aren't taking estrogen. Very few women take cyclic estrogen today.

Continuous Estrogen and Cyclic Progestin

Because estrogen alone has been linked to the development of endometrial (uterine) cancer, women whose uterus is intact need to add progestin (a synthetic form of progesterone) to their HRT program because progestin protects against endometrial cancer. The estrogen–progestin combination appears to eliminate the added risk of endometrial cancer from taking estrogen alone.

Experts may recommend this dosage regimen for women with severe symptoms. With this method you take estrogen every day and add progestin for only part of the month. Because you do take progestin, you will have a period although the periods eventually become light. Some women find this disconcerting. Your menopausal symptoms won't reappear because of the estrogen you're still taking, but you'll still have a period because of the progestin.

Cyclic Estrogen and Progestin

In this scenario you take estrogen on days 1 to 25, adding progestin on days 14 to 25. On day 26, you don't take either hormone, and you will then have a period. The periods eventually become light, but you will bleed. The problem with this method is that your menopausal symptoms may return during the five or six days you're not taking estrogen.

Continuous Estrogen and Progestin

Designed for women who want to avoid having a period, you take both hormones every day (although the progestin is taken in a lower dose). Because there are no days on which you don't take hormones, you don't bleed. The problem with this method is that there may be breakthrough bleeding, so many women prefer the cyclic method so they at least know when the bleeding will occur. Women who do keep taking hormones continuously, however, eventually will stop bleeding after about a year.

Continuous Progestin

If you can't take estrogen, you may want to try just progestin to relieve hot flashes. This hormone won't protect you from heart disease, but it may help you retain bone mass. It is of no use against dryness of vaginal tissue or urinary problems.

Kinds of Hormones

In addition to the dosage regimens from which to choose, there are many different types of hormones.

Estrogens

Premarin

One of the most well-known types of estrogen, this hormone is purified from the urine of pregnant mares and is the most frequently used estrogen in the United States. Typical doses are 0.625 mg and 1.25 mg. Higher doses are available (2.5 mg and 5.0 mg), but they are not often prescribed.

The "conjugated equine estrogens" are absorbed through your intestines, where they are transmuted into estrone and estradiol; when they reach the liver, they arrive in very high concentration, far higher than the dose you would normally produce from your own ovaries. The liver metabolizes the estrogen, which then enters the bloodstream in much lower concentrations.

Premarin can ease vaginal dryness and insomnia, and it is excellent for hot flashes. Although it can decrease bone loss, it doesn't guarantee you won't get osteoporosis; and it may have beneficial effects on your heart. However, there is probably a risk of breast cancer and definitely a risk of endometrial cancer with this hormone.

Side Effects   The most common side effects are breast tenderness and swelling, PMS, rash, facial and body hair growth, pain with contact lenses, migraine, dizziness, headache, depression, changes in libido, increased triglycerides, and blotchy skin. If you take Premarin you won't get a period, although about a quarter of women on this hormone do have occasional bleeding.

Withdrawal   If you choose to stop taking Premarin, you should tell your doctor and taper your dose so you're not suddenly subjected to severe withdrawal symptoms. You can do this by alternating a whole pill with a half pill for two months, or taking a whole pill every other day, dropping down to a half pill every day for two months, then half a pill every other day for two months. Then you can stop.

Some women object to Premarin because they believe that the method of obtaining the mare's urine is inhumane. Pregnant mares are tied in stalls for most of their pregnancy, wearing urine collection harnesses. Critics of this practice say that the harnesses can cause sores and that the horses are sometimes denied water to concentrate their urine (the farmers are paid more for highly concentrated urine). Other women find the idea of taking hormones obtained from a horse to be "unnatural."

17b-Estradiol

The primary form of estrogen that your ovaries produce is 17b-estradiol, which is available both as a skin patch (Estraderm) and as a pill (Estrace). The patch sidesteps conversion by the liver (the oral form is transformed in the liver to a weaker version of estrogen). This form of estrogen is natural in that it's the same chemical formula as the estradiol produced in your own body.

Estrone Conjugate

Estrogen conjugate (Ogen or Ortho EST) is derived from the primary type of hormone produced by the ovaries after menopause. It can both ease symptoms and protect against osteoporosis.

Progestins

Natural progesterone—most like the form we produce in our own body—is available, but it's rarely used because it is plant based and therefore it can't be patented. Instead, manufacturers produce progestin, in which the molecules of natural progesterone have been slightly altered. Although the terms "progesterone" and "progestin" are often interchanged, they are not really the same thing.

When hormone replacement was first introduced, only estrogen was given to patients. But when women taking estrogen began developing uterine cancer, experts realized it was important to add progesterone or progestin at the end of the cycle to induce a menstrual period, shedding the lining of the uterus and minimizing the risk of uterine cancer by preventing a buildup of tissue.

However, progestins have other effects in the body. When combined with estrogen, progestin can worsen bloating, depression, headaches, irritability, fluid retention, breast tenderness, and cramps. They also appear to block some of the other helpful estrogen-related benefits of ERT.

There are several different forms of progesterone and progestin. One brand name for progestin, Provera, is so well known that "Provera" and "progestin" are often used interchangeably. There are other brand names, however, including Curretab, Amen, and Cycrin. Generic Provera is medroxyprogesterone acetate (MPA).

Many women take progestin as a pill, although it is poorly absorbed when taken this way. For this reason you'll need high dosages (200 mg twice a day). Because progesterone can make you sleepy, many women instead take 300 mg right before bedtime, or you can insert the pill into your vagina.

Alternatively, you can take progesterone as vaginal or rectal suppositories twice a day, but they are messy. Newly approved by the FDA is the progesterone ring (Estring). Inserted into the top of the vagina, it gradually releases the hormone for up to three months. It can be easily removed if there is a problem, and it provides constant levels as long as the ring is in place.

Progestin injections are painful and aren't a good choice for hormone replacement therapy.

As of yet, no progestin patch is approved in this country.

Testosterone Replacement

In addition to estrogen and progesterone, your ovaries produce a small amount of male hormones and continue to do so even as the female hormone levels drop. As you enter perimenopause, the levels of male hormones do decrease slightly as well. Many women will never need testosterone replacement, but it may be an important component to your HRT if you have lost your ovaries abruptly or if you are troubled by declining libido.

Testosterone can improve your libido, and decrease anxiety and depression; adding testosterone especially helps women who have had hysterectomies. Testosterone also eases breast tenderness for perimenopausal women who have this problem before their periods and for women who have just started HRT. Testosterone also helps prevent bone loss.

Of course, no treatment is perfect, and testosterone has its side effects. Some women experience mild acne and some facial hair growth, but hormone levels are typically very low and most women don't appear to have extremely masculine changes.

You can take daily testosterone pills (Estratest, a combination of estrogen and testosterone) or alternate testosterone with estrogen every other day. A combination of estradiol and testosterone injections is given every four to six weeks.

Stopping HRT

Doctors, when they recommend HRT at all for perimenopausal women, recommend you only take these hormones for a few years. When you stop, you may notice that some or all of your symptoms return—but it's also possible that you won't notice any symptoms at all because you've passed through that transition time. It's also important to realize, however, that the protective benefits of HRT will also stop when you cease treatment.

Of course, the other question is *when* you should stop taking hormone replacement. If the only reason you're taking HRT is to alleviate your unpleasant symptoms, you can probably taper after two or three years. But if you want to take hormones to protect yourself from osteoporosis, you should probably continue until your bone loss would naturally begin to slow down—usually around age 65. The relationship between estrogen replacement and heart disease is still unclear, although experts seem to believe that you need to keep taking hormones to protect your heart.

In any case, you should never simply stop taking hormones without your physician's knowledge.

Hormones and Symptoms

If you and your doctor do decide to undergo HRT to alleviate your symptoms, it's a good idea to know as much as possible about what sorts of hormones may work best for which symptoms.

Hot Flashes

Hot flashes respond well to most types of estrogen, in either pill, patch, or injection. (Doctors don't usually prescribe estrogen creams for this symptom.) You will want to have the lowest possible dose of estrogen to control the hot flashes.

Because it takes four to six hours for oral estrogen to fully enter the bloodstream, take your medication just before you go to bed. Otherwise, you may still experience problems with night sweats, insomnia, or early morning awakenings. Some women find they do best by taking oral estrogen twice a day, at morning and at night. It should take three to four weeks before you notice relief; if you haven't noticed any easing of hot flashes after three months, your doctor may increase the dosage gradually or choose another route of administration. Women who still have a uterus will also need to take progestogen together with estrogen.

Bleeding

A doctor prescribes hormones to try to balance the hormonal shift that may be the cause of excessive bleeding, but they don't always work the way they are intended. After making sure your bleeding isn't caused by some other medical condition, your doctor will probably prescribe a progestin to balance the estrogen; at the end of the cycle, the lining of the uterus will be shed, and you'll have a period.

If progestin or progesterone doesn't control the bleeding, the doctor may resort to Lupron, a drug that inhibits the hormones from the hypothalamus and triggers a reversible menopause. It usually will stop the bleeding, although not always.

Vaginal Dryness

Estrogen creams (Premarin cream and Estrace) can be applied to the vagina and can be very effective in treating dried, thinning tissues, causing an increase in your blood levels of estrogen. The estradiol in Estrace is very well absorbed from the vagina into your blood and will raise your blood levels of estrogen; Premarin (primarily estrone) is not so well absorbed.

You only need a very low dose of estrogen to treat vaginal dryness with a cream, and it doesn't appear to have any side effects: only 0.1 mg of estrogen is needed to lubricate the vagina. It is particularly important for women with a history of breast cancer to use the lowest dose possible.

The cream is applied inside the vagina every day for up to a month; after that you can apply the cream less often. Applying it daily for longer than six weeks reduces its effectiveness. Micronized progesterone, which will make you sleepy, can also cure insomnia and is recommended to be taken before bedtime for this reason.

Depression

There is no link between menopause and depression, but studies do indicate that taking estrogen and progestin (especially Provera) can cause depression.

Incontinence

Estrogen won't help stress incontinence, but estrogen cream may help if your incontinence is related to vaginal dryness.

Memory/Thinking

Estrogen can help sharpen thinking skills and can be taken from two to four years for this purpose.

Anti-estrogens

Researchers may soon be able to offer women new types of hormone therapy that provide some of the same protection against heart disease and bone loss as estrogen, but without the increased risk of breast cancer. This new class of drugs, known as "anti-estrogens," may be available within the next year or two because three companies (Eli Lilly & Co., Pfizer Inc., and SmithKline Beecham) are racing to be the first to sell the anti-estrogens.

IF YOUR SYMPTOMS DON'T GO AWAY ON HRT . . .

Sometimes hormone replacement doesn't stop all your symptoms. If this is your situation, you can try changing the kind of estrogen you are taking or increasing the dose. Of course, this isn't something you can decide on your own—you need to discuss it with your doctor.

Women who still have problems with hot flashes despite being on hormone replacement may find that adding vitamin E can make the flashes disappear. (Although there has been no solid scientific evidence that vitamin E is effective against hot flashes, many women swear it does help.) If you want to add vitamin E, the usual dose is 400 mg twice a day. Ask your doctor if you can add this amount of vitamin E.

In particular, one anti-estrogen, raloxifene (known technically as a selective estrogen receptor modulator), mimics the effects of estrogen in the bones and blood, but blocks some of its negative effects elsewhere. It's called an anti-estrogen because for a long time these drugs had been used to counter the harmful effects of estrogen that resulted in breast cancer. (For example, the cancer-fighting drug tamoxifen is an anti-estrogen.) But oddly enough, in other parts of the body these drugs mimic estrogen, providing estrogen's protection against heart disease and osteoporosis without putting you at risk for breast cancer.

Like estrogen, raloxifene works by attaching to an estrogen "receptor," much like a key fits into a lock. When the hormone "key" clicks into the receptor "lock," it sends a signal to certain genes in that cell. When raloxifene clicks into the estrogen receptors in the breast and uterus, it blocks estrogen at these sites. This is the secret of its cancer-fighting property. (Many tumors in the breast, for example, are fueled by estrogen; if the estrogen can't get in, then the cancer can't grow.)

There may be other benefits. Preliminary results from a study of more than twelve thousand women suggest that raloxifene increases bone density by up to 3 percent. It also appeared to protect against heart attacks by lowering total cholesterol, LDL ("bad") cholesterol, and fibrinogen.

The potential benefit of taking raloxifene instead of traditional estrogen replacement therapy is that the new drug doesn't cause uterine bleeding, bloating, or breast soreness, side effects that prevent many women from using hormone replacement therapy. Moreover, raloxifene may decrease the risk of breast cancer, which is a relief to women concerned about the potential increased risk of breast and uterine cancer associated with traditional estrogen therapy.

Raloxifene is one of several drugs being designed by scientists to mimic the benefits of estrogen in menopausal women. Researchers are developing drugs that have different effects on specific tissues, unlike hormones that affect many tissues of the body. Eventually, scientists may be able to design drugs to match a particular woman's medical profile.

The concept of designing a drug that has the beneficial effects of estrogen without the deleterious effects is quite possible and highly desirable. But there are a few catches. There is no evidence that raloxifene boosts HDL ("good") cholesterol, and it may worsen hot flashes. For another, doctors are still discovering new benefits of estrogen replacement, and it's not clear if anti-estrogens will be as effective and versatile as estrogen itself. Still, experts are hoping that the new generation of drugs may offer many of the benefits of HRT with fewer risks or side effects.

New Research

However, there are indications that alternatives to hormone replacement may be found in a completely different area of research. Harvard scientists recently have found a way to block the onset of menopause by keeping the cells in the ovaries from dying.

While trying to develop a way to preserve fertility in cancer patients, scientists inadvertently stumbled on two chemicals that can keep the ovaries functioning. The research is still in the experimental stage, but one of the scientists suggested that hormone therapy might become a thing of the past if their technique were refined, because an implant of these chemicals could theoretically preserve ovarian function.

Scientists cautioned that any specific applications of the research at the moment are "strictly speculative."

What's Next?

The next chapter discusses how perimenopause affects libido, as well as how HRT affects it. For those of you who are thinking of getting pregnant—or want to avoid pregnancy—you'll learn about the relationship between perimenopause and fertility.

7 Sex and Fertility

Every woman who is entering perimenopause needs to understand that hormones play a role in psychology and sexuality. It is certainly true that as we age we tend to engage in sex less frequently—and this is true for both men and women. Studies show that the rate of sexual activity falls steadily for both women and men between ages 20 and 40, when the decline then becomes even more dramatic. Still, among women in early menopause, 7 percent of women between age 45 and 50 said they had no interest in sex, rising to 20 percent by age 51, and to 31 percent by age 56.

Physical Changes and Sex

The changes in emotions and interest in sex are only one part of the picture. As you enter perimenopause, you undergo physical changes in your genitals as well. As your ovaries shut down, the levels of estrogen and testosterone drop. It is this loss of testosterone that may be, at least in part, the culprit behind your loss of libido, which is more pronounced in some women than in others.

Testosterone affects libido, but lowered estrogen levels affect the physical makeup of the entire genital area. Some of the first changes you may notice involve the outer genitals, as pubic hair gets thinner and the labia (lips) lose fat tissue. This means that the labia become less sensitive to touch.

When you were younger, during sexual arousal the blood flow out of your genitals slowed down as blood vessels became constricted; this boosted your lubrication and swelling. As you enter perimenopause, blood flow to the genitals slows down. This means that the clitoris, vagina, and other tissues may not become as engorged, which can mean you don't feel quite as sexually aroused. This doesn't affect all women equally, but if it affects you it could interfere with your sexual pleasure.

As you progress through your midlife years, your breasts won't increase as much in size during sex either. When you were younger, sexual arousal caused the blood to rush to the breasts, swelling them by as much as a fourth their former size. At perimenopause, your breasts don't swell as much—and by the time you are postmenopausal, they likely won't swell at all. (However, once you have given birth your breasts won't change in size no matter how young you are.)

Meanwhile, inside the vagina the tissue is becoming thinner and more fragile; left unstimulated by masturbation or intercourse, the walls of the vagina will eventually atrophy as nerves and glands don't get enough blood. As the nerves become impaired, you will experience less sensation during intercourse; as the glands fail, you will lubricate less easily.

At this point sex may well be painful. But if you stop having sex, the situation will only worsen, speeding up the genital deterioration. As time goes on, your vagina will shrink to the point where it's possible to tear the walls of the vagina if the tissue is thin and dry enough.

Skin Changes

The withdrawal of estrogen also creates changes in your skin, which can make you hypersensitive to touch. You may notice that the starched sheets that once felt so good now feel irritating, and that wool that once felt cozy now simply itches. This may be one reason why you no longer feel excited by the way your partner touches certain areas of your skin. As estrogen levels drop, the sensitive nerve endings in your skin change too.

Normal skin sensitivity usually returns if you take hormones. If you can't (or you don't want to), there are other solutions. Be honest with your partner about what feels good and what doesn't, and try to find other areas of the skin that are more responsive.

Rarely, women report a "crawling" sensation on their skin when they get into bed. Known medically as "formication," this disappears with hormone replacement treatment. Although uncommon, it is not a sign that you are crazy or losing interest in your sexual partner.

Vaginal Infections

Other changes may also be taking place. You may notice you have more vaginal infections. They occur because the acid-base balance of the vagina begins to change, and the higher pH level makes the vagina more susceptible to infection. The dry, thin tissue of the vagina is also more likely to become infected and inflamed, leading to itching and discharge.

Lack of Sexual Interest and Hormone Replacement

According to one Yale University study, both men and women have less interest in and respond less readily to sex as they age, and one partner's lack of interest does affect the other. Still, the study found that if you've had a healthy sexual relationship before perimenopause, chances are you can maintain that relationship into old age.

Research clearly shows that it's possible to enjoy your sex life not just through perimenopause, but throughout your menopausal years as well. Indeed, many women develop an increased sexual desire during their early 50s because not having to fear unwanted pregnancies has left them feeling freer.

In addition to psychological reasons, there may be physical reasons for the reinterest in sex after menopause. After menopause, women exhibit a higher testosterone-to-estrogen ratio because estrogen levels fall, whereas testosterone levels stay the same—or even increase. Because testosterone is the hormone responsible for sexual desire, the shifting levels of these hormones mean you have renewed desire as you age.

There are other ways to boost a flagging sexual interest, however. Proponents of hormone replacement point to the fact that many women recover their sexual interest when they begin taking hormones. Studies have shown that up to 90 percent of postmenopausal women regained their normal level of desire once they started HRT.

However, for perimenopausal women who may not be able to take hormone replacement, there are other ways of increasing desire. These include:

- doing Kegel exercises (see Chapter 2)

- applying moisturizers or lubricants to dry vaginal tissues

- practicing visualization or fantasies

- viewing erotic tapes or reading erotic books

Some women who are on HRT report that they still have no interest in sex. This could be because their therapy does not include the male sex hormones (androgens) that govern your sex drive. Some experts are working on adding androgen to HRT, which can improve libido for some women.

However, although this may seem like the perfect answer, androgens also may stimulate male sexual characteristics, such as facial hair, and may interfere with the cardiovascular benefits of taking HRT.

Pregnancy During Perimenopause: Yes or No?

As American women postpone pregnancy, they find they are trying to conceive while their ovaries are gearing down. For other women who assume they can no longer get pregnant, perimenopausal pregnancies can be a surprise.

It may come as a surprise to you that women in their 40s have the second highest rate of unplanned pregnancies and abortions. Most likely, women of this age accidentally get pregnant because they don't realize they are still fertile. It's important to understand that missing a period doesn't mean you have stopped ovulating. It's actually possible to fluctuate between fertility and nonfertility during the perimenopause years, which is why doctors recommend that you keep using contraception for a full year after your last menstrual period.

By the time you reach perimenopause, you still have ten thousand eggs left. All you need is one of those to become fertilized to get pregnant. However, just the fact that you have the eggs doesn't mean they will be released. Your follicle may not release an egg each month; even if it is released, that egg may be at least 40 years old and may no longer be capable of getting fertilized and attaching itself to your uterus.

If you're not sure whether or not you're still fertile, you can take the FSH test to find out. A reading between 20 and 40 means that you are probably in perimenopause, which may indicate it could be more difficult, but not impossible, to get pregnant.

Women on hormone replacement therapy usually won't get pregnant because their ovaries are no longer expelling eggs to be fertilized. However, your doctor will likely warn you to continue using contraception for a year after your last period just in case your ovaries reactivate.

If You Want to Avoid Getting Pregnant

Remember that just because your cycles aren't regular, you're in your late 30s, and you're perimenopausal, you still have between a 30 and 50 percent chance of getting pregnant if you don't use contraception.

In fact, if you still have your ovaries and you're using hormone replacement therapy, the estrogen may actually boost your ovarian function and increase your chances of getting pregnant.

On the other hand, pregnancy that doesn't involve artificial insemination is rare after the age of 50, although it occasionally occurs.

The most common way to avoid pregnancy, which is also the most often used form of contraception in the United States, is sterilization. Birth control pills are also very popular as a contraceptive, especially during the perimenopause. Because oral contraceptives contain estrogen and progesterone, they can help control hot flashes and irregular periods and are often prescribed instead of HRT for this reason. This is why more and more women are choosing to go on the Pill during their 40s, eventually switching to HRT when they enter menopause later in life.

Despite the nagging fear of birth control pills and cancer, for many women the benefits of the Pill outweigh the danger. (Of course, women at high risk, including those who smoke or have blood clots or heart problems, may not want to take birth control pills.) Pregnancy in the 40s is more risky than taking the Pill, especially because perimenopausal women can use the very lowest dosage, as their ovarian function is already suppressed.

Still, many women in their 40s choose a different birth control method from one they might have chosen earlier in their lives. Older women often have heavier or longer periods than they did in their 20s or 30s, for example, so they would not choose an IUD, which can make bleeding even heavier.

Birth Control Pills

Although in the past experts discouraged women over age 40 from using the Pill, today's lower-dose choices make this contraceptive device a better choice for nonsmoking women than in the past. Choosing the Pill won't alter your perimenopause, but it may mask the symptoms.

Intrauterine Devices (IUDs)

This method is normally marketed for older women who are less concerned about infertility because there is a link between IUDs and pelvic inflammatory disease (PID) (and infertility). Because up to 20 percent of women who try an IUD give it up because of excessive bleeding, perimenopausal women who are already suffering from this symptom may want to choose a different method of contraception.

Remember to report any incidence of excessive bleeding to your doctor because this may be related to health problems other than the IUD. Also report any symptoms of lower abdominal pain, fever, chills, cramps, and unusual vaginal discharge (all symptoms of PID).

Barrier Methods

The diaphragm, cervical cap, and condom are the contraceptive methods most often recommended to women in midlife. Used by women in midlife, these methods are extremely reliable. A properly fitted diaphragm is 98 percent effective in preventing pregnancy, or just about as effective as the Pill or the IUD. The condom, used together with contraceptive foam, is almost 100 percent effective.

An added bonus of barrier methods is that the accompanying contraceptive foam, jelly, or cream can increase lubrication, which is often a problem in perimenopausal women. They can also provide some limited protection against sexually transmitted diseases.

Although the diaphragm can still be used by midlife women, certain medical conditions that can occur at this age—prolapsed uterus, fibroids, or protruding bladder—can make it almost impossible to insert a cervical cap or diaphragm. And because perimenopausal women are already prone to urinary tract infections (UTIs), the additional tendency to develop these infections among diaphragm users may make this method an unpopular choice at this stage in your life. If you suspect your diaphragm is playing a role in recurrent UTIS, ask your doctor about getting a slightly smaller diaphragm (and remember to urinate right after having sex).

Natural Methods

None of the "natural" family planning methods (calendar, temperature, or cervical mucus method) are recommended for perimenopausal women because at this point in your life it is often very difficult to determine when you are ovulating. As ovulation becomes more erratic, you will not be secreting as much mucus and it will be much easier to miscalculate.

If You Want to Get Pregnant

In these days of delayed motherhood, it could very well be possible that you've reached your 40s and are just now thinking about becoming a mother. Most doctors will tell you that if you've tried to get pregnant for a year and failed, chances are that something may be wrong. However, if you are over age 35, waiting a year can be much too long. If you decide you want to get pregnant and you're over age 35, and if after six months of unprotected sex you still aren't pregnant, you should schedule a visit to an infertility clinic.

Statistics show that 80 percent of women under age 34 will get pregnant within 10 months of trying; that figure drops to just 40 percent of women over age 40. That doesn't mean that if you're over age 40, you aren't fertile anymore—you still have a good chance of having a baby eventually. It's just that the chance of getting pregnant during any particular cycle is much lower.

This drop in fertility isn't just a woman's problem; only one third of men over age 40 can impregnate their partners within six months, due to a reduced sperm count or sperm motility.

Infertility Exam

If you haven't been able to get pregnant after six months, your doctor will want to examine both you and your partner, starting with physical and sexual histories. Your partner will undergo a semen analysis and you will have a hormone evaluation, followed by a test after sex to study the interaction of your partner's sperm with your cervical mucus. Your doctor will also want to conduct a test to investigate whether or not your fallopian tubes are blocked. Called a "hysterosalpingogram," it involves injecting dye into the uterus to see whether it can enter the fallopian tubes.

If you are nearing 40, your doctor may include a laparoscopy in order to directly observe your uterus and fallopian tubes.

Remember that it is not a matter of being fertile or infertile; many perimenopausal women are "subfertile." If you fall into this category, you must move quickly so that you have as many options as possible to become pregnant.

Infertility Treatment

When all the tests have been finished, your doctor will have a better idea about what is causing the infertility. If the problem lies in the quality of the sperm, your doctor may suggest you consider using donor sperm. If you have endometriosis or your fallopian tubes are blocked, the problem can be treated during laparoscopic surgery.

If the problem is related to a nonfunctioning ovary, however, it may require more complex treatment. Because older women have much less time in which to get pregnant, experts often recommend in vitro fertilization to perimenopausal women because this method has a greater chance of ending in pregnancy. In vitro fertilization using donated eggs is successful more than 40 percent of the time.

At this point you need to assess why you want to become pregnant. Do you focus on simply wanting to be a parent, or do you want to go through the birth experience? Your answer to these questions should determine whether you opt for adoption, or you choose some type of fertilization.

If you want to go through a pregnancy yourself, you have several options for fertilization:

- your own eggs and donor sperm
- your own eggs and your partner's sperm
- donor eggs and your partner's sperm
- donor eggs and donor sperm

Having a Baby

Regardless of the method by which you become fertilized, once you are pregnant you face a new challenge: staying pregnant. As you age, your risk of miscarriage rises. By the time you are in your early 40s, you have a 33 percent risk of spontaneous abortion; women over age 45 are more likely to lose their baby than they are to carry the child to term. The higher the FSH at any age, the greater the chance that you will have a miscarriage.

Even if you don't have a miscarriage, babies of older mothers run an increased risk for a variety of birth defects and chromosome problems. This is why a variety of tests are recommended for all mothers over age 35, including amniocentesis and chorionic villus sampling. Amniocentesis, in which a sample of amniotic fluid is withdrawn and tested in the sixteenth week of pregnancy, is used to screen for genetic disorders. Cvs can diagnose a variety of genetic problems as early as the tenth week of pregnancy.

The good news is that if you manage to get pregnant and the screening tests are all positive, you will likely deliver a healthy baby. A healthy perimenopausal woman with good prenatal care should expect a healthy baby.

What's Next?

As you begin to make your lifestyle choices for the midlife transition, it's a good time to take stock and make sure you're as healthy as possible. In the next chapter you'll read about the best ways to make healthy lifestyle choices—tips for exercise and diet to take you into the second half of your life.

8 Looking and Feeling Your Best: Diet and Exercise

It's important to remember that perimenopause is not a disease—it's just the body's way of getting used to a different level of circulating hormones. If your symptoms are mild, you can often get relief by making the following simple lifestyle changes.

Stop Smoking

There are many reasons to stop smoking, but perimenopause is a good time to focus on quitting. Because smoking causes your blood vessels to constrict, the habit can actually intensify and prolong hot flashes. Moreover, research has shown that smoking can speed up the onset of perimenopause by as much as two years. In addition, smoking increases the risk of heart disease at any age; as you lose estrogen, the risk becomes even greater.

Watch Your Diet

It's a fact that most women gain weight during the perimenopausal years, and the weight gain will continue after menopause (between 10 to 15 pounds after menopause and more if you're already obese).

What you want to aim for at this point in your life is a "good diet"— one that you should have been following all along, but probably weren't. This means no crash diets, but sensible, obvious choices.

There are also a few specific things you can do with food to mitigate the symptoms of perimenopause. Remember that spicy food, caffeine, and alcohol, as well as too much salt or sugar, can trigger hot flashes. Try drinking two 8-ounce glasses of soy milk daily for as long as your symptoms of perimenopause persist. Soy foods (including tofu) contain phytoestrogens—plant-based hormones that replace small amounts of estrogen.

Fiber

A high-fiber diet can lower your risk of colon/rectal cancer and help you control your weight by moving food quickly through the intestinal tract.

We all know that fiber is good, but if you haven't been eating very much and you suddenly decide on a high-fiber diet, you'll be bloated and uncomfortable. The American Institute for Cancer Research recommends that women need between 20 and 35 grams of fiber per day; work up to that amount slowly. Start by adding the fiber foods that are easy to digest, such as fruits and whole-grain bread. Drink at least 8 to 10 cups of water a day, and add beans last.

Fiber can cut down on constipation and keep your digestive tract healthy, and it can also help prevent you from absorbing some fat. (Of course, too *much* fiber isn't healthy either; moderation is the key.)

High-fiber foods include:

- beans (lima, navy, and kidney beans especially)

- bran

- cereals high in fiber (look for 5 grams per serving, and understand that a whole cereal bowl is really at least two servings as listed on the box of cereal)

- fruit

- vegetables

- whole-grain breads

Cut Fat

In the best of all worlds less than 30 percent of your calories should come from fat—those of you who want to lose weight should aim for a diet of less than 20 percent fat. Here's how you can do that:

- Avoid fast food.

- Limit your use of butter, oil, and salad dressings (or switch to nonfat varieties).

- Consume nonfat or low-fat dairy products—skim milk, nonfat frozen yogurt, and so on.

- Replace meat with soup, salad, vegetables, rice, pasta, or fish; if you do eat meat, choose chicken without the skin; limit meat or fish portions to 6 oz per day.

- Understand labels: a food can have no cholesterol but be filled with fat. Avoid food that has more than 3g of fat per 100 calories.

- Trim visible fat and fatty skins before cooking to avoid absorbing fat into the meat.

- Steam, poach, broil, boil, bake, microwave, or grill—don't fry or bake with creamy sauces.

- Snack on fresh fruit, popcorn (no butter added!), pretzels, whole-grain crackers, vegetables.

Cut Down on Sugar

Even if you're not diabetic, too much sugar can interfere with your absorption of minerals and vitamin B complex. Sugar also worsens gum disease and tooth decay, and it can make you more nervous or anxious because of vitamin B depletion.

And although you may not be diabetic at the moment, excess sugar can be a factor in bringing on adult-onset diabetes type II and other blood sugar problems. These conditions can get worse after menopause.

Cut Down on Salt

If you've been feeling bloated, the last thing you want to do is load up on salt, which can make you feel heavy because it retains fluid in the body. Too much salt also boosts blood pressure.

Remember that salt is found not just in your saltshaker, but in most processed foods (such as catsup and canned soups). Read labels and look for low-salt products; herbs or spices can improve flavor just as well.

Because salt is an acquired taste, as you cut down on salt you'll notice that you will probably get used to eating food this way, and very salty foods will be less appealing.

Lose Weight

It's a sad fact that as you age, you need to lower your calories or you'll gain weight. For every decade past your 20th birthday, you need to cut between 2 and 8 percent of your calories. You can offset the need to eat less by boosting your exercise regimen, which will boost your metabolism. If you are more than 30 percent overweight, you're at risk for heart disease, even if you have no other risk factor. It's particularly important to keep fat off your waistline and abdomen—the most dangerous places to put on pounds as far as your heart is concerned.

As you age, your percentage of body fat increases and your lean muscle mass drops. This can be reversed by eating a sensible, low-fat diet and getting enough exercise.

You can reduce the fat in your body by reducing the fat in your diet—it's as simple as that. Instead of reducing your entire calorie consumption, try to cut your fat intake to between 20 and 30 grams a day. (Don't cut all the fat out of your diet, or the lack of fat will affect your skin, hair, and nails.)

Fat-free choices include most vegetables and fruits, grains, and beans. Most fat grams are lurking in dairy products, meats, and fried foods.

Get Your Calcium

If you're experiencing early menopause, you need between 1,000 and 1,500 mg of calcium each day to offset the increased risk of osteoporosis, the bone-thinning disease. Most of us only take in about 500 mg of calcium each day.

Some women like to take antacid tablets, which contain a form of calcium carbonate that can supplement your calcium. Your dosage depends on how much calcium you're getting in your diet. Be sure to check with your doctor if you want to take calcium supplements of any kind. If you do take calcium supplements, it's better to take them with food to boost the absorption of the calcium.

You can easily make sure you're getting the right amount by drinking three 8-ounce glasses of low-fat milk each day. If you can't stand that much milk, try eating a diet rich in calcium:

- green vegetables (broccoli, kale, turnip, collard, mustard, dandelion)—but not spinach, which *inhibits* the absorption of calcium by the body

- tofu (choose the kind that's set in calcium caseinate)

- shellfish

- canned salmon (with bones)

- sardines

- mackerel

- calcium-fortified orange juice (contains as much calcium as milk)

- yogurt (8 oz contains 300 mg of calcium)

- cheese (2 oz contains 300 mg of calcium)

CALCIUM ALERT

It's not enough to take in plenty of calcium. You also need to be aware of the many drugs and other substances that can leach calcium from your bones. The following items can lead to calcium deficiency, either by interfering with calcium absorption or boosting its excretion:

- alcohol (two drinks per day or less)
- caffeine
- cholestyramine
- Metamucil
- nicotine
- processed foods
- excess protein (more than 40 grams per day)
- sodas (contain both caffeine and phosphorus, which are particularly depleting)
- tetracycline

WHAT TO LOOK FOR IN A CALCIUM SUPPLEMENT

If you don't get enough calcium in your diet, you need a calcium supplement. Look for the words "calcium carbonate" on the ingredients list. Either generic or supermarket brands are fine, and you can also choose calcium carbonate antacids (such as Tums). Don't take more than 500 mg of calcium at a time (that's the amount your body can best absorb). Remember to take supplements with meals because there is some evidence that it is better absorbed when your stomach is secreting acid.

Take Your Vitamins

Vitamins are a good idea at any time of your life, but they make particular sense when you're dealing with perimenopause because you're likely facing stress from fluctuating hormones. Nutritionists recommend that to get enough dietary vitamins perimenopausal women should take calcium, vitamin D, iron, and vitamin B$_6$ in addition to eating a diet rich in fruits and vegetables. If you do choose to take extra vitamins or minerals, it's important to discuss them with your doctor or a qualified nutritionist. Getting the right dose is extremely important, and overdosing can have toxic effects.

Antioxidants

Of all the vitamins you can take, antioxidants are probably the best ones to focus on as you're dealing with aging. As long as you're looking at your diet, remember that one way to lower your risk of cancer and heart disease is to be sure to consume antioxidants—vitamins A, C, and E. As your body burns fuel for energy, it releases toxic substances called "free radicals," a dangerously mutant form of oxygen. Free radicals travel through your body helping to digest your dinner and battle your infections, but unchecked they can swell to lethal numbers. The level of antioxidants in your body rises with every puff of a cigarette, each belch from a smokestack, and every minute of excessive exposure to sunlight.

Antioxidants pick up the free radicals before they can enter your organs, and they help your body excrete them. Studies have not proven just how much antioxidants can do, but they certainly aren't harmful taken in normal amounts. It's also true that the average American doesn't get enough antioxidants by eating foods that contain them—yellow and green vegetables, citrus fruits, and wheat.

To boost your body's ability to cope with free radicals, try taking vitamins A, C, E, B$_1$ (thiamine), B$_6$ (pyridoxine), and B$_5$ (pantothenic acid). Of these, A, B, and E have a direct impact on the perimenopausal changes going on in your body. Vitamin E is probably the best when it comes to neutralizing the free radicals before they do any damage, reducing tissue damage after inflammation or a heart attack, and increasing resistance to cancer cells. (However, if you *have* cancer, you may want to avoid vitamin E because one Swedish study found that women with breast cancer did not respond to treatment as well if they took vitamin E.)

Vitamin A

Vitamin A and carotenoids (in green and yellow vegetables) can help decrease the risk of heart attacks and strokes, may cut lung cancer risk in smokers, and are important for vision. You can find vitamin A in carrots, spinach, collard greens, beet greens, mustard greens, squash, broccoli, let-tuce, peaches, apricots, cantaloupe, papaya, and sweet potatoes. Fish oils (cod liver oil) contain retinol (vitamin A). For a supplement, women need about 5,000 IU of vitamin A and 3 to 5 mg of betacarotene daily. Do *not* take more than this. Taking estrogen supplements may also increase your need for this vitamin because high estrogen levels have been shown to interfere with vitamin A's ability to function in the body. You should *never* take more than 20,000 IU of vitamin A daily. Too much can lead to headaches, hair loss, blurry vision, emotional problems, and so on.

Vitamin B Complex

The group of B vitamins all play a key role in keeping you healthy as you approach menopause. Many women who have taken birth control pills or who are on hormone replacement are deficient in vitamin B. Symptoms of deficiency include depression, fatigue, concentration problems, loss of libido, and insomnia. In fact, some experts believe that the more severe hot flashes some women get when they stop taking estrogen occur because the hormones had depleted their folic acid. Synthetic hormones can deplete vitamin B, which is responsible, among other things, for stabilizing the chemistry of the brain.

The vitamin B complex is considered to be an "antistress" compound, and includes vitamin B_1 (thiamine), B_2 (riboflavin), B_3 (niacin), B_5 (pantothenic acid), B_6 (pyridoxine), and B_{12} (cyanocobalamin).

Experts have suspected for a long time that vitamin B_6 may ease perimenopause symptoms because it acts as a diuretic, but no studies have yet come up with any solid evidence. Some studies have found that a deficiency of B_6 may be linked to anxiety or irritability.

To achieve the best balance, you should probably take the B vitamins together as "vitamin B complex," and if you're over age 40, you need to be sure you're getting at least 100 mg of niacin. Don't take more than 25 mg of vitamin B_6; more can lead to tingling and burning sensations.

Fortunately, the B vitamins are usually found all together in foods. The best sources include whole breads and cereals, oatmeal, dried beans, brewer's yeast (except for B_{12}), liver, nuts, eggs, and seeds.

Folic acid. Helps you manufacture and use estrogen, and helps form healthy red blood cells.

Niacin. Helps your body produce estrogen and other sex hormones while cutting cholesterol and dilating blood vessels. Niacin may be prescribed to help reduce preperiod headaches.

Pyridoxine (B_6). This natural diuretic helps fight bloating and possibly other premenstrual symptoms. It also interacts with estrogen in ways that are still not fully understood.

Riboflavin (B_2). Important in the release and activity of a variety of hormones (including estrogen) and helps keep skin, nails, and hair healthy.

Thiamine (B_1). Keeps the vagina (and other mucous membranes) healthy.

Vitamin C

Another antistress vitamin, vitamin C, has calming effects and can help heal wounds, maintain collagen, and ease excessive bleeding. It works together with vitamins A and E to boost the immune system and acts as a powerful antioxidant.

Experts disagree about how much of this vitamin you need for optimum health, ranging from 250 mg to 1,000 mg. You can get vitamin C in citrus fruits, tomatoes, broccoli, peppers, celery, cauliflower, kiwifruit, and cantaloupe. You need at least two fruits or glasses of juice a day, plus at least one vegetable from the preceding list. If you're not getting that much, think about taking a 500-mg supplement.

Vitamin D

Although vitamin D is not an antioxidant, it is of great importance to perimenopausal women because it can help your body absorb calcium, keeping your bones strong. You usually get enough vitamin D simply by being outdoors in the sun. Indeed about 75 percent of the vitamin D in your body is produced in the skin with the aid of ultraviolet radiation from the sun. Otherwise, the best way to get enough vitamin D is to eat plenty of salmon (the best source), followed by mackerel, sardines, and tuna. Butter, eggs, and fortified milk also provide vitamin D. Most multivitamins contain the required 400 IU of vitamin D you need. Remember that too much vitamin D can cause bone *loss*; don't take more than 1,000 units per day.

New research also suggests that vitamin D may play a role in cutting your risk of breast cancer because cancer survivors with a vitamin D receptor in their breast tissue survived longer than those women without such receptors. Researchers at the University of California, San Diego, have linked a decreased incidence of breast cancer to living in areas that receive more exposure to ultraviolet light. Conversely, cities with the lowest amounts of ultraviolet light had the highest concentrations of breast cancer.

Vitamin E

There is no conclusive scientific proof that vitamin E can do a thing for your hot flashes. Still, many women insist that vitamin E in fact has helped lessen the problems of this unpleasant perimenopausal symptom. Some studies have not found vitamin E is more effective than placebo; others indicate the opposite. Scientists do know that vitamin E is essential to the proper functioning of blood and for the production of sex hormones—so this may have something to do with its success in taking the heat out of hot flashes.

Herbalists advise 400 units twice a day, up to 1,200 units—far more than the 100 units recommended by the FDA. Because extremely large doses of vitamin E can cause muscle weakness and fatigue, it's probably not a good idea to take more than 1,000 mg a day.

Although vegetable oil, nuts, whole grains, and wheat germ are the best sources of this vitamin, you'll need supplements to get 1,000 units every day.

The best sources of vitamin E in your diet are:

- whole-grain cereals and breads (including brown rice and millet)

- lettuce, peas, asparagus, cucumber, and kale

- dried beans

- unprocessed vegetable oils (wheat germ, corn, safflower, sesame, peanut, and soybean oil)

- fish (haddock, herring, and mackerel)

- lamb and liver

- mango

Do NOT *exceed 1,000 IU per day without consulting a qualified nutritionist. If you develop blurred vision while taking vitamin E, discontinue the supplements immediately. Women with high blood pressure, diabetes, or rheumatic heart disease, or those who take digitalis, should consult a doctor before taking this vitamin.*

Some experts recommend adding a B-complex supplement, 500 mg of vitamin C, and 25 mcg of the mineral selenium to boost the effectiveness of vitamin E.

Iron

You won't need an iron supplement unless you have an iron deficiency. The best way to take a supplement is by taking ferrous sulfate with a glass of orange juice and a little food; this helps you absorb the iron and lessens the chance of an upset stomach. It may take up to three weeks of taking iron supplements before you feel better, but you may need to continue the treatment for up to a year in order to restore your levels of iron.

On the other hand, too much iron can be toxic and can lead to cirrhosis of the liver. This is why you shouldn't take iron supplements unless you have an iron deficiency.

BEST WAY TO TAKE YOUR VITAMINS

You can take a multivitamin, or you can take individual supplements. Keep these tips in mind:

- Check the expiration date (vitamins lose potency quickly).

- Take supplements three times a day, not all at once; water-soluble vitamins have a better chance of being absorbed this way.

- In legal terms the word "natural" means that a vitamin contains a minimum of 10 percent natural ingredients.

- Take a balanced supplement with vitamins *and* minerals.

Exercise

The lack of physical exercise is a real risk factor in a variety of diseases; for example, not exercising is almost as strong a risk factor in heart disease as smoking! Far too many women don't get enough exercise, which would improve not just the heart, but bones, muscles, balance, and weight. Of particular interest for women facing perimenopause, some women report that they have fewer hot flashes when they exercise regularly. Exercise also promotes better sleep and improves mood. A brisk 30-minute, two-mile walk can boost your circulation and increase your tolerance for those almost-inevitable hot flashes.

Of course, when you start out on an exercise program, you need to take into consideration your medical problems and your fitness goals. If you're just starting an exercise program, you should check with your doctor first to make sure your anticipated level of activity is appropriate.

Ideally, you should perform aerobic exercise for 20 to 30 minutes each day—walking, running, cross-country skiing, tennis, swimming. Whatever you choose, select something you enjoy doing; you'll be more likely to stick with it that way. Try to exercise three times a week for 20 minutes, and then gradually increase both intensity and duration. Remember: a little exercise is still better than none. If you can't commit to a three-day-a-week exercise schedule, don't give up on the idea of exercise completely.

In addition, you can benefit from twice-a-week weight-lifting workouts to make your muscles strong and keep your bones dense; workouts also boost muscle mass, which will raise metabolism and help you burn more calories. According to the American College of Sports Medicine, you should try eight to twelve repetitions each of 8 to 10 exercises at each session.

No matter which exercise you choose, you're going to have to exercise fast enough and long enough to get your heart rate up. You can judge how hard your heart is working by measuring how fast your heart beats during workouts. To do this, you'll need to figure out your "maximum heart rate" and your "target heart rate range."

Finding Your Maximum Heart Rate

Your maximum heart rate is a lot like the top speed of your car—the maximum heart rate is the most it should ever be, not the rate your heart *should* be working when you exercise. It's not hard to figure out. Just subtract your age from 220. If you're 40, here's what you do:

$$
\begin{array}{r}
220 \\
- \ 40 \\
\hline
180 \text{ beats per minute}
\end{array}
$$

Your maximum heart rate is 180 beats per minute.

Target Heart Rate Range

Now that you know your maximum heart rate, it's not hard to figure out your target heart rate range—this is the heartbeat that you're aiming for when you exercise. The target heart rate range is 70 to 85 percent of the maximum heart rate. For example, if you're 40, you would calculate as follows:

1. Take your maximum heart rate (180 beats per minute).

2. Multiply 0.70 times 180 = 126 beats per minute.

3. Multiply 0.85 times 180 = 153 beats per minute.

When you exercise, you'll want your pulse to be somewhere between 126 and 153 beats per minute the whole time. It's a good idea to start out exercising lightly, so that your heart rate stays in the lower part of your heart rate range. This way you'll be able to keep going for the full 20 or 30 minutes. As you become more experienced, you can do more strenuous exercising that will boost your heart rate into the higher ranges.

Drink Plenty of Water

The more you sweat (and the more you bleed, if you're still having irregular or heavy periods), the more fluid you lose. Be sure to drink at least eight 8-ounce glasses of water a day.

Fluids you might want to watch out for, however, are those that contain caffeine. This powerful stimulant may make you feel alert, but during perimenopause it can worsen your mood swings and breast tenderness. It also can interfere with your absorption of calcium and iron. Those women with problems of insomnia may find that caffeine worsens sleeplessness as well. Remember, however, that if you quit drinking coffee and cola drinks suddenly, you're likely to go through withdrawal-related headaches, irritability, nervousness, and so on. Try lowering your daily caffeine level gradually, or switch to half-caffeinated, half-decaffeinated beverages until you wean yourself off caffeine completely.

Relax

Deep breathing can give you a feeling of control over your body. Many of the annoying symptoms of perimenopause can be worsened by stress; if you can learn how to relax, you'll feel much better and be less bothered by moodiness, irritability, headaches, and so on. When you know how to relax your body, you'll automatically reduce the harmful effects of stress. And being able to stay calm in the face of stress can provide you with a real sense of self-control.

There are different approaches to relaxation training, from simple relaxation strategies to standard meditational visualization. When you relax or meditate, you focus on something besides stressful thoughts for a period of time. This rests your mind, channeling it away from dwelling on stress-causing problems. As you relax or meditate, your body has time to recuperate. Withdrawing from problems and calming your mind can calm your body, blunting the adrenaline surge of stress.

When you do relaxation exercises or meditate regularly, here's what happens to your body:

- Breathing slows.

- Blood pressure drops.

- Muscles relax.

- Anxiety lessens.

- Stressful thoughts disappear.

- Irritability eases.

- Stress headaches disappear.

- Thinking becomes clearer.

- Focus and concentration improve.

You might find it helpful to build a relaxation or meditation time into every day, a time when you can look forward to relaxing. Ideally, you'll notice fewer hassles with stress if you can manage to do this every day.

Some people like to start off the day with a meditation or relaxation period of about 20 minutes; others like to use it to unwind after a rough day.

How to Meditate

Before you can begin to meditate, you need to be able to relax your body. You'll probably be surprised at how much tension you find in your muscles. Until you relax them, you may not have realized how rigid some of those muscles were.

Here's how to take the first step:

1. Find a position that feels comfortable, either sitting or lying down.

2. Close your eyes.

3. Relax your arms with hands slightly folded on your lap.

4. Begin taking slow, deep breaths.

5. Breathe rhythmically from the abdomen, not the chest.

6. As you say the word "relax" silently to yourself, focus on the muscles at the top of the head and consciously relax them.

7. When you feel the top of your head seem to relax, move down to the eye area. Keep repeating "relax" as you consciously focus on each muscle group.

8. Don't move on until you can feel that area relax.

9. Move on to the sinus area of your face, and *relax*.

10. Move to the muscles of your ears and the back of your neck. Here is the seat of quite a lot of tension, so spend some time here. Don't move on until you can actually feel those muscles loosen.

11. Move on down all the way to your toes, relaxing each section of your body.

This is just one very effective way of relaxing your muscles. If you're enjoying this feeling, and you'd like to know more, you could take yourself to a deeper state of relaxation with meditation or self-hypnosis. There are different ways to relax, of course.

Deeper Meditation

Now that you've learned how to enter a state of light relaxation, you can experiment with meditation, a deeper state of relaxation.

1. Follow the preceding steps to relax your body.

2. Focus on your breathing. As you breathe out, silently repeat a word or a phrase (such as "om" or "peace").

3. When thoughts pop into your head, let them go calmly. Return to your word.

4. Continue for 10 or 15 minutes at first; you may wish to extend your meditation as you become more experienced.

After several weeks of practice, most people say they feel not just more relaxed after meditating, but more likely to stay calm in response to stress.

Visualization

Visualization is a more active procedure than meditation, and it may be easier to accomplish, because you are actually *doing* something with your mind. Basically, visualization involves relaxing yourself and then imagining a calming scene. The principle behind visualization and imagery is that you can use your mind to re-create a relaxing place. The more intensely you call up the scene in your mind, the stronger and more realistic the experience will be. In "active visualization" you can give yourself suggestions while you're in the scene, called "affirmations."

1. Go through a total body relaxation, as just discussed.

2. When you have fully relaxed, still with eyes closed, imagine a calm, beautiful scene in full detail. You can pick a place that you've already visited or make one up. This may take practice; some people are gifted visualizers, and others find this more difficult.

3. Don't just visualize a picture; listen to the wind blow. Smell the scent of new-mown hay. Feel the spray of the surf.

4. Still with your eyes closed and while you're in the scene, give yourself a positive affirmation: "I feel peaceful" or "I feel completely relaxed in every social situation."

5. Keep the affirmations positive. Don't say "I want to stop feeling miserable and stressed"; say "I will feel pleasantly relaxed and calm in every situation."

6. At the end of the visualization, tell yourself "When I open my eyes, I will feel calm, peaceful, and completely refreshed." Then open your eyes, and prepare to be amazed!

What's Next?

Now that you've learned how to make the most of your midyears by eating well and exercising, it's time to talk about how to make the rest of your life as healthy as possible. In the next chapter we'll discuss a health plan for life, including all the tests you need and when and how to take steps today to head off the "big three" diseases facing perimenopausal women—heart disease, breast cancer, and osteoporosis.

9

Preventing Heart Disease, Osteoporosis, and Breast Cancer

Midlife is the best time not only to find out about the symptoms of perimenopause, but also to focus on other aspects of your health as well because many health problems begin at this point in a woman's life. Learning about prevention now can help you head off significant health problems later.

By the age of 45, all women should schedule a "perimenopausal visit" with a physician to discuss menopause and get some health counseling and disease risk assessment. In fact, this is the perfect time to get an overall health evaluation, including a complete checkup, mammogram, breast exam, Pap smear, fecal occult blood test, cholesterol measurements, FSH test, cardiogram, and possibly a bone density measurement.

Unfortunately, many women feel slightly ridiculous going in for a wide range of tests when they feel perfectly healthy. But doctors say that the best way to ensure that you stay healthy is to start taking care of yourself before serious problems begin.

Medical History

When you're at the doctor's office for a checkup and complete physical exam, the first thing a good doctor will do is to take your personal and family medical history. The doctor will want to know if you have a history of:

- cancer (especially immediate family with breast, ovarian, or uterine cancer)
- diabetes (type I or type II)
- heart disease
- liver disease
- osteoporosis
- pregnancy
- surgery

The doctor will also want information on:

- allergies (especially drug allergies)
- diet
- exercise regimen
- medications you take
- menstrual cycle pattern
- smoking or substance abuse
- weight

Then the doctor may well discuss the following tests with you, many of which you should definitely schedule at this point in your life.

Blood Pressure

You should have your blood pressure taken every other year from age 30 on up. Continual blood pressure checks are extremely important because high blood pressure is one of the most treatable causes of stroke. High blood pressure is also an important factor in heart disease.

Bone Density Test

There are several kinds of tests you can take to measure your bone density. These reliable, painless tests don't take much time and can usually be finished within 30 minutes. In many testing centers you don't even have to change into an examination robe.

Standard X-rays can't really determine bone mineral density—you'd have to lose about 25 percent of your bone before an X-ray would pick up the deterioration.

The two best and most common tests today for bone density are the dual-energy X-ray absorptiometry and the dual-photon absorptiometry, used primarily to test bone in the hip and spine.

The dual-energy X-ray absorptiometry (DEXA) test measures current bone mineral content at hip, spine, and/or wrist, the most common sites of fractures caused by osteoporosis. At the moment, there are about 700 DEXA machines in the United States. In much the same way as a baseline mammogram is used, this test can establish a basic reading for your bone health against which your doctor can measure future tests. The DEXA can help show whether you are losing or building bone mass—or just staying the same.

Your bone density is compared with two standards, known as "age matched" and "young normal." The age-matched reading compares your bone density with what is expected in someone of your age, sex, and size. The "young normal" reading compares your bone density with the estimated peak bone density of a healthy young adult of the same sex. Generally, the lower your bone density, the higher your risk for a fracture.

Not every woman needs this 20-minute test. For example, it wouldn't reveal much bone loss to most women in their 30s, unless a woman was experiencing early menopause or sustained unexplained fractures. Guidelines suggest that the test should be done for women who take corticosteroids, women who have had a cracked or fractured vertebra detected on X-ray, women who have hyperparathyroidism, or women in menopause who are considering hormone replacement therapy. In the test, you lie fully clothed on a table as the scanner passes above you emitting radiation only ½0 of what is contained in a chest X-ray.

Alternatively, you can check for bone density with an ultrasonogram of your heel, which is reported to be just as accurate in predicting hip fractures, according to some researchers at the University of California at San Francisco. Ultrasound is much faster and less expensive than densitometry and is radiation free.

Two other tests include the CAT scan and the single-photon densitometry, both of which are used to evaluate bones in the wrist. You can also get a lab test that checks the amount of calcium in your urine. It's also a good idea to keep track of your height. If you notice a decrease, consult your health care practitioner.

There is a significant range of cost for these tests, and not all insurance companies will pay for them. For example, the dual-photon test can range from $50 to $250 and up, depending on where in the country the test is done.

Unfortunately, of the 20 million American women with osteoporosis, 80 percent (that's 16 million) have no idea they have the disease. Efforts to increase the rate of diagnosis are accelerating. In 1995 there were only a thousand diagnostic sites in the country with machines that could measure bone density. By 1997 there were more than four thousand sites.

FIND A BONE DENSITY TESTING SITE

To find the nearest testing center, call the National Osteoporosis Foundation Action Line: (800) 464-6700.

Blood Pressure and Cholesterol

These tests can check for the risk of cardiovascular disease. Because estrogen protects the heart, younger women have a lower risk of heart disease than do men. As menopause nears, however, the risk of heart disease in women rises sharply.

Like high blood pressure, high cholesterol is often a forerunner to heart disease. Middle-aged women with normal cholesterol levels are encouraged to have their levels checked every five years.

Breast Cancer Check

Mammograms to check for the presence of breast cancer should be scheduled after your doctor does a breast exam. Mammography is a low-dose X-ray technique used to examine the breast. A baseline mammogram should be done by age 35, so that a normal X-ray can be used to compare future mammograms, even when there is no reason to believe there is a lump or cyst.

Special equipment and specially trained technicians perform mammography. Be sure that the facility you use is approved by the FDA-regulated system created by the American College of Radiology. Radiologists who read mammograms must undergo special training in mammography.

When getting your mammogram, you should undress above the waist so the technologist can position your breast between two plastic plates. The plates are then pressed together to flatten the breast tissue. It is not painless—there is some discomfort, but it is not unbearable and lasts for just a few seconds. Some women may experience sore breasts for a day or two afterward.

A typical screening includes two views of each breast (one from above, and one from the side). Normally, the technician examines the pictures immediately to determine if further X-rays are needed or whether an ultrasound may be required. If anything irregular is detected—a mass, asymmetry, changes from earlier mammograms, abnormalities of the skin, or enlargement of the lymph nodes, further testing may be recommended. This could include an ultrasound of the breast, a biopsy or needle sampling, or consultation with a breast surgeon.

Women at high risk of breast cancer who are over age 40 may want to schedule a mammogram every year. Otherwise, you should have a mammogram every one to two years until age 50, and after that you should have one every year.

For questions about mammography or to locate a center near you, call the National Cancer Institute's toll-free Cancer Information Service at (800) 4-CANCER.

In addition, you should check your own breasts each month (at the same time each month) to learn what is normal for you. Any changes should be immediately brought to the attention of your doctor.

Cholesterol Measurement

This blood test should be done every one to two years, depending on your family history. The test results are very important in being able to predict heart disease.

Electrocardiogram

It's a good idea to have a baseline ECG done in your 30s and another done at age 45 to check the health of your heart.

Eye Exam

You should schedule your eye exams at least every five years (unless you have problems before then) until age 50. Thereafter you should have an eye screening every four years. Eye exams should include a test that screens for glaucoma.

Fecal Occult Blood Test

This test, which checks for cancer, should be done every other year until age 50, when it should be done every year.

Pap Smears

A Pap smear is a screening test your doctor can use to check for precancer of the cervix (the opening to your uterus). Only half of all American women over 40 are getting a regular Pap smear, despite the fact that older women are more likely to die from this condition than are younger women.

Before Pap smears were available, cancer of the cervix was a common and often deadly cancer; today, cervical cancer is rare and easily treated in women who undergo regular testing.

The test isn't usually painful and won't take more than a few moments. Your doctor will insert a speculum into the vagina to spread the vaginal walls apart; then a soft brush is rubbed against the cervix to scrape off some cells. These cells are placed on a glass slide, stained with a special dye, and checked under a microscope. At the same time many doctors do an exam to check the uterus and ovaries, plus a breast exam.

Before your Pap smear:

- don't douche for three days before the exam

- don't have sex or use tampons, birth control foams, or jellies for five days before the exam

- take showers, not tub baths, for 48 hours before the exam

- tell the doctor if you have signs of infection (discharge or itching); these problems may need to be treated before your Pap smear

Most medical experts recommend that all women have a yearly Pap smear to check for cervical, uterine, or endometrial cancer; it is especially important if you have multiple sexual partners or you have certain diseases (such as herpes type II).

An abnormal result may mean cancer, but it also may simply be the result of many different changes that can take place on the cervix. Pap smears may be abnormal if the cervix is inflamed or irritated.

Alternatively, the cervix may be going through a change called "dysplasia." This means that cells on the smear look abnormal under the microscope. Dysplasia is *not* the same thing as cancer, although it may lead to cancer if not properly treated.

If you have had three consecutive normal Pap smears, you may want to discuss with your doctor whether you can have a Pap smear performed only every other year.

Pelvic Exam

Your gynecologist will do a pelvic exam every other year from age 20 to 39 and every year after age 40 to check for ovarian and uterine tumors, cysts, and cancer. It is usually done together with a Pap smear.

If any cysts or tumors are found, your physician may recommend a pelvic ultrasound, which helps distinguish between the two. A third test—the CA 125 blood test—can help detect or at least verify ovarian cancer, although its accuracy is not high.

Sigmoidoscopy

This procedure is usually done in the doctor's office for an inspection of the last 12 inches of the large intestine. It should be done about every four years after age 50.

The Big Three: Heart Disease, Breast Cancer, and Osteoporosis

Ask any group of women which disease they fear the most, and chances are they'll tell you it's breast cancer. Yet despite this widespread concern, the real killer that is far more deadly is almost ignored by women and is too often overlooked by their physicians—heart disease. For some reason most women hardly give the third serious disease they face in midlife—osteo-porosis—a moment's thought. And yet osteoporosis can rob women not just of their mobility, but their independence. The perimenopausal period is the perfect time to take stock of your health and make certain that you are well protected against these three killers.

Heart Disease

Heart disease is the number one killer of American women, accounting for almost half of all female deaths in this country. Despite common misinformation, women are eight times more likely to die of a heart attack than from breast cancer.

Women rarely have a heart attack before menopause because of the protection that estrogen offers against the blood vessel blockage. Studies suggest that estrogen increases the "good" cholesterol (HDL) and decreases "bad" cholesterol (LDL) in the blood. One of the best ways to protect yourself against heart problems is to keep close tabs on your blood pressure. Hypertension often carries no symptoms, but it can lead to stroke and heart disease before you ever realize there is a problem. This is why regular blood pressure screenings are an essential part of any preventive health care plan. Doctors also recommend an electrocardiogram (a tracing of the electrical activity of the heart) by age 45.

Risk Factors

A woman who smokes is two to six times more likely to have a heart attack than someone who doesn't. Women who smoke and also take birth control pills with both estrogen and progesterone are at special risk. But if she stops smoking, no matter how long or how much she had smoked, her risk of heart disease drops rapidly. Other risk factors include:

- advanced age
- having a close relative that had a heart attack or stroke before age 60
- physical inactivity
- high blood pressure
- high cholesterol or triglycerides

- diabetes
- drinking more than three alcoholic drinks daily
- being overweight
- stress

The Solution

In the *New England Journal of Medicine* (October 24, 1989, issue), research-ers at Brigham and Women's Hospital and Harvard Medical School write, "Postmenopausal women who take estrogen generally have lower rates of cardiovascular disease than women of similar age who do not." The research was part of the ongoing Harvard Nurses Study of more than 120,000 nurses, yet many doctors will agree that the use of estrogen replacement to prevent heart disease in postmenopausal women is still open to debate. Some experts estimate that women on estrogen replace-ment therapy can halve their risk of heart disease.

If you're not sure about hormone replacement, there is a host of lifestyle changes you can make to decrease your risk of heart disease. These include watching your blood pressure, learning how to handle stress, eating a healthy, low-fat diet, and keeping track of your cholesterol and triglycerides. You'll want to get plenty of exercise—at least 30 min-utes of aerobic exercise three times a week. Of course, quitting smoking is one of the single most powerful ways you can cut your risk of heart disease.

Osteoporosis

Somewhere between ages 30 and 35 a woman accumulates the highest amount of bone mass she will ever have. After age 35, however, bone den-sity begins to decrease. Osteoporosis is more common among women than stroke, heart attack, and breast cancer *combined*—yet women over age 50 still may not fully understand how they can maintain their bone health.

Women are at special risk for osteoporosis because they typically have lighter frames than do men, so they have less bone mass to start with. They also may be at risk due to their higher rate of depression because depression may increase a woman's risk for broken bones, according to an October 1997 study by scientists at the National Institute of Mental Health. They found that the hip bone mineral density of women with a history of major depression was 10 to 15 percent lower than normal for their age—so low, in fact, that their risk of hip fracture rose by 40 percent over 10 years. The affected women (average age of 41) had bone loss equivalent to that of a 70-year-old woman.

Experts suspected the link between bone loss and depression might be due to the women's higher levels of the stress hormone cortisol. Excess cortisol levels—a common feature of some depression—is also known to cause bone loss.

The Problem

Osteoporosis ("porous bone") is the most common and debilitating bone disorder in the world. It is characterized by loss of bone mass, which makes your bones thin, brittle, and prone to fractures. Osteoporosis today affects 25 million Americans and is not usually diagnosed until a fracture occurs (usually in the spine, hip, or wrist).

Although many women think of bone as a sort of dead, hardened substance, bone is, in fact, living tissue that is constantly renewing itself. In the prime of your life, there is a healthy balance between bone tissue that is being produced and tissue that is being resorbed.

In your teen years, you actually build more bone than you lose; by about age 35, the balance begins to change and you start to lose more bone than you can replace. Most people lose about 1 percent of their bones per year. When you enter perimenopause, however, you begin to lose bone faster, and by the time you are menopausal, your loss rate is about 3 percent a year in each of the first five years after menopause ends.

Risk Factors

Women with two or more risk factors should have an osteoporosis evaluation during their perimenopause years. You are at higher risk of developing osteoporosis if you:

- have a family history of the disease

- had an early menopause (either natural or surgical)

- are Caucasian or Asian

- lead a sedentary lifestyle

- don't get enough calcium in your diet

- are thin and/or have a small frame

- use alcohol heavily

- smoke

- have anorexia or bulimia

- use corticosteroids and anticonvulsants

- are depressed

Prevention

Fortunately, osteoporosis is not inevitable. Women in their 40s can minimize bone loss and decrease their fracture risk by eating healthy meals and getting enough exercise. There are a number of other things you can do to head off osteoporosis:

- Start adopting a healthy lifestyle *today.*

- Work on weight-bearing exercises three times a week.

- Eat foods high in calcium (take supplements as well).

- Avoid alcohol, which can reduce your ability to retain calcium.

- Quit smoking, which can hasten menopause.

- Consider HRT early in perimenopause to head off the development of osteoporosis.

- Avoid excessive amounts of protein and sodium, both of which can significantly increase calcium loss.

New Treatment

Although there is no cure for osteoporosis once it occurs, several different drugs can be used to treat the disease and sometimes reverse its course. These include:

- estrogen (to block bone loss)

- calcitonin (a nonestrogen treatment that blocks bone loss)

- Fosamax (a potent new nonestrogen treatment that blocks bone loss and may decrease fracture risk)

Fosamax (alendronate), which was approved by the FDA several years ago to treat osteoporosis, was cleared in April 1997 for preventing the disease as well—the only drug other than estrogen approved to prevent osteoporosis. Because not all women want to, or can, take estrogen, Fosamax can be helpful in preventing osteoporosis.

According to studies, women who received Fosamax increased their bone mass in spine, hips, and total body after two years on the drug. Experts suggest that women could have their bones tested, and if their bone mass was below the standard level, they would be candidates for preventive use of the drug.

New drugs known as anti-estrogens developed to treat osteoporosis may soon be on the market. The drug likely to be approved first is Eli Lilly's raloxifene (Evista), followed by droloxifene (Pfizer). Drug companies Glaxo Wellcome PLC, SmithKline Beecham PLC, and Zeneca PLC are all researching their own compounds. There is some concern, however, that little is known about the long-term effects of these drugs. Some critics note that the new drugs are related to the cancer-fighting drug tamoxifen, a drug that has been linked to uterine cancer (for more information see Chapter 6).

ONE SERVING OF CALCIUM
(20% OF DAILY REQUIREMENT)

- 1 c skim or low-fat milk

- 1 c low-fat or nonfat yogurt

- 1 c calcium-fortified juice

- ½ oz cheese

- 3 oz canned sardines with bones

Breast Cancer

As you age, your risk of developing breast cancer—no matter what your family history—rises dramatically. The breast cancer risk of a 25-year-old woman is only 1 out of 19,608. But by age 40 your risk increases to 1 in 217; by age 45 it is 1 in 93. Moreover, your risk continues to rise the older you get.

Despite the controversy about the cost effectiveness of mammograms for women in their 40s, most doctors agree with the current American Cancer Society guidelines that recommend screening mammograms every year or two for women in the 40 to 49 age group and every year after age 50 (provided you don't have a history of breast cancer).

Risk Factors

There are a number of risk factors for the development of breast cancer. At the moment, one out of every nine women in our country will develop breast cancer sometime in her lifetime. Risk factors include:

- a family history of breast cancer in first-degree relatives (mother or sister)

- early menarche (beginning of menstruation)

- first child after age 40

- no children

- fibrocystic disease

In addition, some studies suggest that high-fat diets, bottlefeeding instead of breastfeeding, or using alcohol may contribute to the risk profile.

Some studies have also found that for certain women, the use of HRT may contribute to the development of breast cancer. However, these findings are by no means accepted uncritically.

However, it is important to realize that although having several risk factors may boost your chances of having breast cancer, the interplay of factors is complex. The best way to assess your personal risk for breast cancer is by seeking a consultation for a risk assessment at one of the many breast cancer centers located throughout the United States.

The Solution

There is no sure way to prevent breast cancer other than prophylactic mastectomy—and even that may not prevent breast cancer from appearing in the chest wall beneath the breast. At the moment, mammography remains the best way of detecting signs of breast cancer early.

Today, studies have shown that conservative treatment—a lumpectomy, or partial mastectomy—offers the same odds of survival as does a total mastectomy in women whose breast tumor is small and has not infiltrated the lymph nodes. New studies suggest that a combination of chemotherapy and radiation for women who undergo lumpectomy offers the best chance of long-term survival.

Organizations Concerned with Perimenopause

American Association of Naturopathic Physicians
2366 Eastlake Ave. East, Ste. 322
Seattle, WA 98102
(206) 324-8230
Offers a list of licensed naturopaths around the country ($5).

American Association of Retired Persons (AARP) Women's Initiative
601 East St. NW
Washington, DC 20049
(800) 424-3410
Has a free fact sheet about hormone replacement therapy.

American College of Obstetricians and Gynecologists
409 12th St. SW
Washington, DC 20024
(202) 638-5577
Provides three free pamphlets (send self-addressed, stamped envelope) about estrogen, osteoporosis, and menopause. Also offers a listing of physicians in your area.

American Fertility Society
1209 Montgomery Hwy.
Birmingham, AL 35216
(205) 978-5000
Provides a list of reproductive endocrinologists in addition to information on infertility during the perimenopausal period.

American Heart Association
7320 Greenville Ave.
Dallas, TX 75231
(214) 373-6300
Provides the latest information about heart disease, perimenopause, and HRT. Check the phone book for the local chapter nearest you.

American Holistic Medical Association
4101 Lake Boone Trail, Ste. 201
Raleigh, NC 27607
(919) 787-5181
Publishes a national directory of medical doctors who use alternative treatments ($5).

American Menopause Foundation, Inc.
Empire State Bldg.
350 Fifth Ave., Ste. 2822
New York, NY 10118
(212) 714-2398
An independent nonprofit foundation interested in research, education, advocacy, and support of women in menopause. They operate a national network of support groups that deal with alternative treatments (among other issues).

American Reproductive Health Professionals
2401 Pennsylvania Ave. NW, Ste. 350
Washington, DC 20037
(202) 723-7374
Provides a free copy of a brochure on perimenopause.

Association of Women's Health, Obstetric and Neonatal Nurses
700 14th St. NW, Ste. 600
Washington, DC 20005
(202) 662-1600

Biofeedback Society of America
10200 West 44th Ave.
Wheat Ridge, CO 80033
(303) 420-2902; (303) 422-8436
Offers guidance about where to find a biofeedback center or a qualified practitioner, as well as general information on the types of problems that can be improved using this technique.

Boston Women's Health Book Collective
465 Mt. Auburn St.
Watertown, MA 02172
(617) 625-0271
A nonprofit organization devoted to women's health education, offering health-related materials through its Women's Health Information Center.

CHOICE
Concern for Health Options, Information, Care and Education
125 South 9th St., Ste. 603
Philadelphia, PA 19107
(215) 985-3355

Federation of Feminist Women's Health Centers
633 East 11th Ave.
Eugene, OR 97401
(503) 344-0966

Financial District Women's Health Services
582 Market St., Ste. 100
San Francisco, CA 94104
(415) 982-0707
Provides midlife counseling and medical referrals.

Herb Research Foundation
1007 Pearl St., Ste. 200
Boulder, CO 80302
(303) 449-2265
Will supply information packets on specific herbs for $7 each.

Hysterectomy Educational Resources and Services Foundation (HERS)
422 Bryn Mawr Ave.
Bala Cynwyd, PA 19004
(215) 667-7757
An organization that provides information and counseling for women considering a hysterectomy or who have already had one. Publishes a quarterly newsletter and sponsors conferences around the country.

International Center for Research on Women
1717 Massachusetts Ave. NW, Ste. 302
Washington, DC 20036
(202) 797-0007

International Foundation for Homeopathy
2366 East Lake E., No. 301
Seattle, WA 98102
(206) 324-8230
Provides information on finding a homeopathic practitioner.

International Women's Health Coalition
24 East 21st St., Fifth Floor
New York, NY 10010
(212) 979-8500

Melpomene Institute for Women's Health Research
1010 University Ave.
St. Paul, MN 55104
(612) 642-1951
Since 1981 the institute has focused on the link between physical activity and women's health. At present they are researching the link between menopause and exercise. Annual membership fee includes the *Melpomene Journal* three times a year.

National Alliance of Breast Cancer Organizations
1180 Avenue of the Americas
New York, NY 10036
(212) 719-0154
A clearinghouse for many of the groups offering information on prevention and treatment of breast cancer.

National Breast Cancer Coalition
1707 L St., Ste. 1060
Washington, DC 20036
(202) 296-7477

National Center for Homeopathy
1500 Massachusetts Ave. NW
Washington, DC 20005
(202) 223-6182
Provides nationwide directory of practitioners and homeopathy study groups, sponsors conferences, and offers information on finding a homeopathic practitioner in your area ($6).

National Institute on Aging Information Center
P.O. Box 8057
Gaithersburg, MD 20898
(800) 222-2225
Has free information on menopause, exercise, and nutrition.

National Osteoporosis Foundation
1150 17th St. NW, Ste. 500
Washington, DC 20036
(202) 223-2226; (800) 464-6700 action line
Action line can provide the bone mass testing center nearest you. Foundation also publishes a booklet called *Boning Up*, available by mail ($1), and providing information on diagnostic procedures, calcium, exercise, and the latest research.

National Self-Help Clearinghouse
33 West 42nd St.
New York, NY 10036
(212) 840-1259
Offers referrals to support groups and publishes a self-help newsletter.

National Women's Health Network
1325 G St. NW
Washington, DC 20005
(202) 347-1140
A national public-interest organization dedicated to women and health, sponsoring many educational and research projects. The organization has published a booklet on hormone replacement therapy and offers a newsletter, *The Network News*. A packet of resource material costs $5.

National Women's Health Resource Center
1440 M St. NW, Ste. 325
Washington, DC 20037
(202) 293-6045

North American Menopause Society
P.O. Box 94527
Cleveland, OH 44101
(216) 844-8748
A group that offers a mainstream perspective on menopause treatment, with lists of suggested readings and physicians in your area who specialize

in menopause. Answers written questions for information about menopause, and publishes a medical journal.

Office on Women's Health
Office of the Assistant Secretary for Health
200 Independence Ave. SW
Washington, DC 20201
(202) 690-7650

OWL (Older Women's League)
730 11th St. NW, Ste. 300
Washington, DC 20001
(202) 783-6686
A politically active group that lobbies for equal opportunities for midlife women, with local chapters nationwide that provide referrals to support groups. Publishes a bimonthly newspaper, *The Owl Observer*.

Planned Parenthood Federation of America, Inc.
810 Seventh Ave.
New York, NY 10019
Offers the booklet *Menopause: Another Change in Life* and other helpful brochures ($3). Also offers counseling and gynecological care.

Resources for Midlife and Older Women
226 East 70th St., Ste. 1C
New York, NY 10021
(212) 439-1913
A nonprofit social service agency for midlife and older women that offers quick information and medical/psychological referrals. Also offers referrals to agencies providing services such as personal financial management, legal rights, employment, and so on.

Santa Fe Health Education Project
P.O. Box 577
Santa Fe, NM 87504
Provides information on research and educational services.

Society for the Advancement of Women's Health Research
1920 L St. NW
Washington, DC 20036
(202) 223-8224

Transitions for Health
621 Southwest Alder, Ste. 900
Portland, OR 97205
(800) 888-6814
Has a free mail-order catalog of natural health care products for midlife women.

United Soybean Board
P.O. Box 419200
St. Louis, MO 63141
(800) 825-5769
Provides information about incorporating soybeans into your diet to ease perimenopausal symptoms.

Wellness Community
2200 Colorado Ave.
Santa Monica, CA 90404
(310) 453-2200
Offers free support groups.

Wellspring for Women
(303) 443-0321
Offers phone consultations with licensed nurse practitioners who can answer questions about conventional hormone therapy, herbal remedies, and natural hormones, and can put you in touch with doctors who can prescribe them. A 45-minute consultation costs $120.

Women's Action Alliance
370 Lexington Ave., Rm. 603
New York, NY 10017
(212) 532-8330
Provides referrals for women in midlife.

Women's Health America Group
429 Gammon Place
P.O. Box 259641
Madison, WI 53725
(800) 558-7046
E-mail: *wha@womenshealth.com*

Women's Health Initiative
Federal Bldg., Rm. 6A09
7550 Wisconsin Ave.
Bethesda, MD 20892
(800) 54-WOMEN

Women's Helpline (NOW, NYC Service Fund)
15 West 18th St., Ninth Floor
New York, NY 10011
(212) 989-7230

Provides referrals to midlife women's groups and services.

Y-Me National Breast Cancer Organization
212 West Van Buren St.
Chicago, IL 60607
(312) 986-8228; (800) 221-2141

Breast cancer information and support group.

Websites of Interest to Women in Perimenopause

Menopause
Helpful site with links to related issues.
http://www.howdyneighbor.com/menopaus/

Menopause Online
A helpful site with lots of perimenopause-related information and links to related sites.
http://www.menopause-online.com/links.htm

Meno Times
An on-line journal dedicated to menopause and osteoporosis.
http://www.aimnet.com/~hyperion/meno/menotimes.index.html

North American Menopause Society
Helpful information with frequently asked questions, links to other sites.
http://www.menopause.org/

Planned Parenthood Federation of America, Inc.
Offers a booklet about menopause that can be downloaded.
http://www.ppfa.org/ppfa/menopub.html

Power Surge Reading Room
An on-line menopause discussion room with an electronic newsletter. It can be accessed in its entirety through America Online with the keyword "Women" followed by the "well-being" icon. It can be accessed in part via the World Wide Web at
http://members.aol.com/dearest/news.htm

Women's Health
A basic site with links to information on menopause.
http://woen.shn.net/index.html

Women's Health Initiative
http://www.nih.gov/od/odp/whi

Menopause Clinics

If you wish, you may seek specialized care at any of the menopause clinics staffed by doctors and nurses with expertise in perimenopausal symptoms. Physicians are board certified in reproductive endocrinology or obstetrics/gynecology. There may also be specialists in human sexuality and psychiatry available as well.

California

Menopause Center at UCLA
Center for Health Sciences, Department of Obstetrics and Gynecology
Rm. 22-177 CHS
1083 LeConte
Los Angeles, CA 90024
(213) 825-7755

Menopause Clinic
University of San Diego Medical Center
3969 Fourth Ave.
San Diego, CA 92103
(619) 294-6130 (clinic phone); (619) 453-3210 (hot flash phone, where a nurse will give you immediate help)

Connecticut

Menopause Clinic
Yale University, School of Medicine
Physicians Building
800 Howard Ave.
New Haven, CT 06510
(203) 785-4708

Florida
Climacteric Clinic
Women's Medical and Diagnostic Center
222 Southwest 36 Terrace, Ste. C
University of Florida
Gainesville, FL 32607
(904) 372-5600

Illinois
Menopause Clinic
University of Illinois Hospital and Clinics
840 South Wood, Rm. 200
Chicago, IL 60608
(312) 996-6870

Northwest Memorial Faculty Foundation
Department of Reproductive Endocrinology
680 North Lake Shore Dr., Ste. 810
Chicago, IL 60611
(312) 908-7269

Massachusetts
Menopause Clinic
Brigham & Women's Hospital
Fertility, Endocrine & Menopause Unit
75 Francis St.
Boston, MA 02115
(617) 732-4220

New Jersey
UMDNJ–Robert Wood Johnson Medical School
Department of Obstetrics and Gynecology
1 Robert Wood Johnson Place—CN19
New Brunswick, NJ 08903-0019
(210) 937-7633

Ohio
Cleveland Menopause Clinic
Mt. Sinai Medical Center
29001 Cedar Rd., Ste. 600
Lyndhurst, OH 44124
(216) 442-4747

Texas
Menopausal Section
Department of Obstetrics and Gynecology
Baylor University
6550 Fannin St.
Houston, TX 77030
(713) 798-7500

Washington, DC
Menopause Care Center
George Washington University
2300 I St. NW
Washington, DC 20037
(202) 994-5656

Publications About Perimenopause and Menopause

A Friend Indeed
P.O. Box 1710
Champlain, NY 12919
$30 per year for ten issues; devoted to the informal discussion of women in menopause or midlife.

Harvard Women's Health Watch
164 Longwood Ave.
Boston, MA 02115
(800) 829-5921
Monthly, $24 per year.

Health After 50
P.O. Box 420179
Palm Coast, FL 32142
(940) 446-4675
$28 per year.

Hot Flash Newsletter for Midlife and Older Women
National Action Forum for Middle and Older Women
P.O. Box 816
Stony Brook, NY 11790
(212) 725-8627
Quarterly publication ($4 per issue; $25 yearly).

Melpomene Journal
Melpomene Institute for Women's Health Research
1010 University Ave.
St. Paul, MN 55104
(612) 642-1951
Annual membership fee includes the *Melpomene Journal* three times a year.

Menopause Management
Carrington Communications, Inc.
P.O. Box 658
Flanders, NJ 07836
(201) 584-3040
Bimonthly, $65 per year.

Menopause News
2074 Union St.
San Francisco, CA 94123
(415) 567-2368
$23 per year.

Midlife Woman
5129 Logan Ave. South
Minneapolis, MN 55419
(800) 886-4354; (612) 925-0020
Bimonthly newsletter, $25 per year; provides practical, easy-to-read articles on health and related topics of interest to women in midlife and beyond.

The Network News
National Women's Health Network
1325 G St. NW
Washington, DC 20005
(202) 347-1140

The OWL Observer
OWL (Older Women's League)
730 11th St. NW, Ste. 300
Washington, DC 20001
(202) 783-6686
Bimonthly newspaper.

Via: A Guide Through Menopause and Beyond
Carrington Communications, Inc.
P.O. Box 658
Flanders, NJ 07836
Quarterly, $19.97 per year.

Glossary

absorptiometry (single- and dual-photo) Two special X-rays that can detect osteoporosis. In these tests, radioactive iodine is injected into the bone and scanned with one or two beams from radioactive sources.

adenomyosis A condition characterized by pieces of the uterine lining imbedding in the walls of the uterus, causing heavy bleeding. In severe cases a hysterectomy must be performed.

adrenal cortex Outer part of the adrenal gland that secretes cortisone-like hormones.

adrenal glands Hormone-producing glands located above the ovaries (one over each kidney) that supply estrogen, progesterone, adrenaline, and androgens (testosterone).

adrenaline A neurotransmitter produced by the adrenal glands that is released in response to fear, emotion, or stress.

amenorrhea The failure to menstruate.

amino acid An organic compound that is considered to be the building block of protein.

anabolic steroids Drugs of the cortisone family that build up tissue. They are sometimes abused by athletes to enhance their performance.

androstenedione A weak androgen secreted by the adrenal glands and menopausal ovaries. It is a major source of estrogen during and after menopause.

anemia Low red-blood-cell count. In women it is often secondary to heavy periods.

anovulatory A term associated with the lack of ripening and releasing of an egg from the ovary. Anovulatory menstrual periods are often irregular and heavy.

antioxidant A substance that prevents oxidation or inhibits reactions promoted by oxygen.

atherosclerosis Thickening of the walls of the arteries, primarily composed of fat.

Bartholin's glands The two glands located on either side of the vagina that secrete mucus, which helps to provide lubrication during sex.

basal body temperature The temperature taken immediately after waking up, before any activity, often used to determine ovulation. The BBT rises as progesterone rises (such as after ovulation).

basal metabolic rate (BMR) Speed at which the body burns its food. A person with a high BMR tends to be thin.

beta blockers A family of drugs that block the activity of adrenaline, used primarily to slow the heart rate and lower blood pressure.

bioflavonoid A constituent of the vitamin C complex.

biopsy A sample; as a verb, it means to take a sample. A biopsy is often used to determine if a tissue is cancerous.

birth control pills Oral contraceptives containing estrogen and progesterone that suppress the release of an egg by the ovary, thus preventing pregnancy.

blood-sugar level The amount of sugar (glucose) circulating in the bloodstream.

breakthrough bleeding Bleeding between periods, usually associated with low-dose birth control pills. Breakthrough bleeding can be annoying, but it is rarely harmful.

calcitonin A "calcium-sparing" hormone released by the parathyroid, thyroid, and thymus glands that slows the breakdown of bone by increasing the amount of calcium and phosphate deposited on bones.

calcium A mineral carried in the blood that is needed to build bones and teeth.

carcinoma in situ A very localized cancer that has not yet penetrated the basement membrane.

carotene A compound found in plants that the body converts into vitamin A.

CBC The abbreviation for "complete blood count," including white and red blood cells.

cervix The rounded narrow lower end of the uterus that is about an inch long and extends into the vagina; it opens during labor to release the fetus.

climacteric The time frame during which a woman passes from her reproductive to her postmenopausal years. It is marked by the gradual waning of reproductive function. It is a more inclusive term than either perimenopause or menopause; means "top rung of the ladder."

collagen A protein that holds many cells together, much like glue. Softer than bone, it supports the skin and other structures.

colposcope A giant microscope used to examine and magnify the cervix and vulva. It is used to help diagnose precancerous and cancerous conditions of the cervix, vagina, and vulva.

colposcopy A diagnostic technique using a sophisticated binocular-like instrument to examine the cervix and vagina and to take a tissue biopsy when a Pap smear has indicated a possible abnormality.

cone biopsy A surgical procedure in which a cone-shaped wedge of tissue is removed from the cervix in order to diagnose and treat cervical precancerous or malignant conditions.

corpus luteum Latin term meaning "yellow body," this is the cyst that forms in the ovary after ovulation. The cells of the corpus luteum produce progesterone and estrogen, in addition to other hormones, and prepare the uterine lining to receive a fertilized egg.

corticosteroids Drugs that resemble the adrenal hormones.

cortisone Adrenal hormone that can be harmful to bones. Synthetic cortisone is a drug that resembles the adrenal hormone.

cryosurgery Freezing. It is usually used in gynecology to treat genital warts and premalignant conditions of the cervix. It is also known as cryotherapy.

curettage Scraping. It usually refers to scraping the uterine cavity.

cystitis Inflammation of the bladder that usually causes frequent and burning urination.

D&C Abbreviation for "dilation and curettage," this term describes a procedure in which the cervix is dilated so that a curette can be inserted into the uterus to scrape the uterine lining. The cells that have been removed are examined under a microscope. The technique is both a treatment as well as a diagnostic tool in the search for a cause of a woman's excessive, dysfunctional bleeding. Often, a D&C stops this abnormal bleeding.

DEXA The abbreviation for "dual energy X-ray absorptiometry," a technique used to measure bone density.

diuretic An agent that triggers the kidneys to excrete water, increasing urine output.

dopamine An important brain neurotransmitter that plays a role in body movement, motivation, primitive drives, sexual behavior, emotions, and immune system function.

dysmenorrhea Painful menstruation.

dyspareunia Painful sexual intercourse.

endocrine glands Ductless glands that manufacture hormones and release them into the bloodstream. The primary endocrine glands include the pituitary, thyroid, parathyroid, adrenals, and ovaries and testes.

endometriosis A painful disease where cells from the lining of the uterus are not shed during menstruation but instead attach themselves outside the uterus or other organs in the pelvic cavity. Difficult to diagnose, endometriosis can cause infertility. The tissue may be found anywhere in the pelvis besides the outside of the uterus, including near the bladder or bowel, or even, though rarely, as far away as the lungs.

endometrium The lining of the uterus that is composed of glandular tissue.

endorphins Chemicals known as the body's "natural" opiates that control pain and emotions and lessen stress, among other things. They are often released during exercise.

enzyme A protein capable of producing or accelerating a specific biochemical reaction at body temperature.

ERT Estrogen replacement therapy. Given to women in menopause to replace the hormones they are no longer producing.

Estrace A form of estrogen that is a pure product of the same estrogen found in the ovaries (17b-estradiol). Estrace is stronger than estriol, and its safety for women at risk for breast cancer is uncertain.

estradiol The primary, strongest estrogen produced by the ovaries. It is produced in large amounts before menopause. Estradiol is most stimulating to the breast tissue.

estriol A form of estrogen that is produced in large quantities during pregnancy. In more than one study, estriol inhibited the spread of cancerous cells in the breast, indicating that it may actually slow down or prevent cancer.

estrogen A class of female sex hormones found in both men and women (but that occur in larger amounts in women). Estrogen is produced by the ovaries and released by the follicles as they mature, and it is primarily responsible for the development and maintenance of female sex characteristics and reproductive functions in women. Estrogen stimulates and triggers a response from at least 300 tissues, and may help some types of breast cancer to grow. After menopause, production of the hormone gradually stops.

estrogen receptors Receptors on the surface of tissues to which estrogen can attach.

estrone A weak form of estrogen derived from estradiol that is naturally present after menopause, when the adrenal glands help the ovaries secrete androstenedione and then convert it to estrone. Fat cells also convert androgens to estrone, so the more weight you carry the more estrones you produce and the less severe your perimenopausal symptoms. Estrone is believed to be more carcinogenic than estradiol.

fallopian tubes Narrow tubes that are attached to the uterus in which fertilization occurs. They are the conduits for eggs to proceed from the ovary into the uterus.

fibroadenoma Usually refers to a solid but noncancerous breast growth often seen in women with fibrocystic breast changes.

fibroid tumors Fibrous, nonmalignant growths most often found in or on the uterus that may grow as big as a grapefruit, pressing on other organs.

follicle A small, round sac; in the ovary, each egg is contained in a follicle.

follicle-stimulating hormone (FSH) The pituitary hormone that stimulates the ovary to mature follicles for ovulation. FSH is associated with rising estrogen production throughout the cycle; an elevated FSH (above 40) indicates menopause has begun.

formication A creeping sensation on the skin, as if it's crawling with bugs. Sometimes occurs in perimenopausal or menopausal women.

free radicals Highly reactive harmful molecular fragments produced during cell metabolism that are thought to be associated with aging, among other things.

FSH See Follicle-Stimulating Hormone.

gamma-linolenic acid (GLA) An essential fatty acid used by the body to produce certain prostaglandins that control several important body processes.

glucose A simple sugar found in the bloodstream.

glycogen The primary form in which carbohydrates are stored in the body for conversion into energy, mostly found in the liver and muscle tissue.

GnRH See Gonadotropin-Releasing Hormone.

GnRH agonists Chemicals that act like GnRH but actually cause the pituitary to make less FSH, eventually decreasing estrogen production.

gonad The ovary or testis.

gonadotropin-releasing hormone (GnRH) One of the hormones that is secreted by the hypothalamus that directs the pituitary to produce gonadotropins (FSH and LH).

gonadotropins The collective term for FSH and LH.

HDL cholesterol High-density lipoprotein. A type of cholesterol sometimes called "good" cholesterol because high levels of it are believed to protect against heart disease. HDL helps keep fat cells from building up on the walls of your arteries.

hematocrit The percentage of blood volume that is composed of red blood cells. A normal hematocrit count for a woman ranges between 38 and 42.

hemoglobin count A measure of the number of red blood cells in the blood. A normal hemoglobin count for a woman ranges between 12 and 14.

histamine A compound found in many tissues that is responsible for the increased permeability of blood vessels and that plays a major role in allergic reactions.

hormone A chemical messenger secreted by a gland that is released into the blood and that travels to distant cells where it exerts an effect.

hormone replacement therapy (HRT) Replacement of both hormones estrogen and progesterone; ERT (estrogen replacement therapy) refers simply to the replacement of estrogen. Women who have had a hysterectomy are almost always given HRT, not ERT, to protect them from endometrial hyperplasia.

hot flash A wave of heat that is one of the most common perimenopausal symptoms, triggered by the hypothalamus's response to estrogen withdrawal.

hyperplasia Excessive tissue growth which is usually benign but, if left unchecked, can sometimes become malignant.

hypoglycemia Low or falling concentration of glucose in the blood, often caused by eating food containing too many carbohydrates.

hypotensive Blood pressure lower than 90/60.

hypothalamus A part of the brain located on top of the pituitary gland that controls much of the hormonal activity of the body, including temperature, sleep, and water balance.

hysterectomy The surgical removal of the uterus. A "radical" hysterectomy includes the removal of the uterus, cervix, ovaries, egg tubes, and sometimes the lymph nodes near the ovaries. A "complete" hysterectomy is the removal of the tubes and ovaries in addition to the uterus. In a "total" hysterectomy the surgeon removes the uterus and cervix, but not the ovaries. In a "subtotal" hysterectomy only the uterus is removed.

incompetent cervix A weakened neck of the uterus (cervix), which during pregnancy allows the cervix to dilate long before it is supposed to. This condition is often associated with miscarriage in the second trimester.

incontinence Involuntary loss of urine or stool. Stress incontinence is characterized by leakage of urine when coughing, when laughing, or during sex and is related to lower estrogen levels. Happens to some perimenopausal women.

insulin A protein hormone secreted by the pancreas into the blood that regulates carbohydrate, fat, and protein metabolism.

in vitro fertilization The fertilization of an egg by sperm in a lab dish or test tube, followed by placing the embryo into a woman's uterus.

Kegel exercises A series of special exercises involving contraction of the muscles around the urethra, bladder, and rectum to improve control of urination or sexual enjoyment.

labia majora The major lips of skin of the female external genitals found on either side of the entrance to the vagina.

laparoscope A narrow metal tube, inserted into the abdominal cavity, that allows a look inside the abdomen and pelvis. It can be used to operate without making a large incision.

laparoscopy A surgical procedure using a long, thin telescope to view the internal organs through a very small incision.

LAVH Laparoscopically assisted vaginal hysterectomy.

LDL cholesterol Low-density lipoprotein ("bad" cholesterol). Associated with a high risk of heart disease due to the accumulation of fatty deposits on artery walls.

LH See Luteinizing Hormone.

luteal phase The part of the menstrual cycle beginning at ovulation and continuing until the onset of the next menstrual period.

luteinizing hormone (LH) A chemical produced by the pituitary that leads to egg maturation and release by the ovary. A surge of this hormone in each menstrual cycle occurs 12 to 24 hours before ovulation.

menarche The onset of menstrual periods at puberty.

menopause The cessation of menstrual periods.

menorrhagia Heavy loss of blood during menstrual periods.

myomectomy Surgical removal of a fibroid from the uterus.

myometrium The muscular wall of the uterus.

neurotransmitter A chemical messenger released by nerve cells in the brain or peripheral nerves to communicate with other nerve cells.

Oestrogel A 17b-estradiol in gel formulation that is rubbed on the abdomen, inner thighs, or back of the arms. Available only in Europe.

oophorectomy The removal of the ovaries (also called an ovariectomy).

osteoporosis Thinning of the bone due to loss of calcium. This disease of chronic bone loss can lead to fractures, difficulty in healing broken bones, compressed vertebrae, pain, and shortened stature.

ovaries The female sex organs where eggs mature, are stored, and then are released. They are the primary source of estrogen in the body.

ovulation The process during which a mature egg is released from the ovary each month.

oxalates Compounds that interfere with the absorption of calcium. They are found in some leafy green vegetables (such as spinach).

pancreas Large organ that extends across the upper abdomen, close to the liver, that secretes digestive juices into the intestinal tract. The juices contain enzymes that act upon protein, fat, and carbohydrates. The pancreas also secretes the hormone insulin directly into the blood.

PAP smear A test used to screen for cervical cancer named for Dr. George Papanicolaou. In the test, a doctor takes a swab of cells from the cervix and vagina that are then examined microscopically.

parathyroid hormone Parathyroid hormone is synthesized and released by the parathyroid glands and controls the distribution of calcium to the bones.

perimenopausal Referring to the time "around the menopause" or "before the menopause" that describes the period when ovarian function and hormone production are declining but have not yet totally stopped.

perineum The structure that contains the outlets of the urethra, the vagina, and the rectum.

pessary A device (usually rubber) that is placed in the vagina and used to support sagging structures of the vagina, uterus, or bladder.

phytoestrogens Plant estrogens.

pituitary gland Also known as the "master gland," this small oval organ is found at the base of the brain behind the bridge of the nose. It produces hormones (including FSH and LH) that regulate the activity of most of the glands. Pituitary hormones also stimulate the ovaries to release estrogen and progesterone.

placebo A pill having no medicinal value often used as a "control" in a research study.

PMS The abbreviation for premenstrual syndrome, a condition experienced by about 10 percent of all women who are extremely sensitive to hormonal change (especially after ovulation).

polyps Soft benign growths with stems that are most often found in organs such as the uterus and rectum. They are usually not malignant, but they can cause a discharge or bleed when irritated.

progesterone The hormone that is produced by the ovary after ovulation, responsible for the changes in the endometrium during the second half of the cycle. Progesterone also prepares the endometrium for implantation and the development of the placenta after implantation.

progestin A synthetic hormone with progesterone-like effects, often administered together with estrogen in hormone replacement therapy.

progestogen A synthetic hormone with the same characteristics as natural progesterone.

prolactin A hormone made by the pituitary gland that stimulates secretion of breast milk. High prolactin levels in nonpregnant women may be an indication of infertility.

prostaglandins A family of hormones formed from essential fatty acids in the uterus and other organs. Prostaglandins stimulate the activity of smooth muscle, including the uterine wall. A type of prostaglandin is related to muscular contractions during labor and menstrual cramps.

reproductive endocrinology The study of the hormonal regulation of reproduction and the menstrual cycle.

serotonin A chemical produced in the brain and found in many tissues (especially the blood and nerve tissue) that stimulates a variety of smooth muscles and nerves. As a neurotransmitter, serotonin is related to mood, emotion, sleep, and other basic functions.

steroids A family of chemicals whose structure and formation come from cholesterol.

supracervical A term that means "above the cervix." It refers to a hysterectomy where the body of the uterus (the fundus) is removed but the cervix is left in place.

surgical menopause The condition in which a woman experiences menopausal symptoms because of a hysterectomy or oophorectomy.

TAH and BSO Total abdominal hysterectomy and bilateral salpingo-oophorectomy.

testosterone Male hormone produced by the testes and in small amounts by the ovaries. Testosterone is responsible for some masculine secondary sex characteristics such as the growth of body hair and a deepening of the voice.

thyroid gland An organ at the base of the neck primarily responsible for regulating the rate of metabolism.

transdermal patch A round plastic patch filled with medicine that is applied to the abdomen, back, or buttocks. In estrogen replacement therapy, the patch contains estrogen and is put on twice a week to administer estrogen. This way the estrogen bypasses the liver and may cause fewer side effects than oral regimens of estrogen.

tubal ligation A surgical method of contraception in which the ends of the fallopian tubes are tied so the egg can't travel from the ovary to the uterus. Also known as "having the tubes tied."

ultrasound A diagnostic tool that uses sound waves (not X-rays) to examine the inside of the body. These procedures are basically risk-free and do not involve exposure to radiation. They are often used to determine if a mass is solid or fluid-filled (i.e., a cyst).

unopposed HRT Hormone replacement therapy containing only estrogen (without progesterone).

ureter The tube that carries urine from the kidney to the bladder.

urethra The canal leading from the bladder to carry urine out of the body.

uterine prolapse A condition in which the uterus slips down into the vagina. In severe cases it protrudes from the body.

uterus A female organ composed of smooth muscle and glandular lining. Also known as the womb.

vagina The muscular canal in the female that extends from the vulva to the cervix.

vaginal atrophy The drying and thinning of the vaginal walls because of loss of estrogen.

vaginitis Inflammation of the vagina.

vestibular vulvitis A painful but basically harmless condition of the outlet of the vagina associated with non-yeast and nonbacterial inflammation.

vulva The tissue surrounding the opening of the vagina, composed of the major and minor lips (labia majora and minora) and the clitoris.

vulvitis Inflammation of the vulva.

Bibliography

Adami, H. O., and Persson, I. Hormone replacement and breast cancer: A remaining controversy? *Journal of the American Medical Association* 274 (1995): 178–79.

Adlercreutz, H., Gorbach, S., and Goldin, B. Estrogen metabolism and excretion in Oriental and Caucasian women. *Journal of the National Cancer Institute* 86/14 (1994): 1076–82.

Anderson, Eric. Ask the doctor: Can soy limit hot flashes? *Medical Tribune News Service*, April 8, 1997.

Barbach, Lonnie. *The Pause*. New York: Penguin Group, 1993.

Barrett-Connor, E., and Kritz-Silverstein, M. Estrogen replacement therapy and cognitive function in older women. *Journal of the American Medical Association* 260 (1993): 2637–41.

Berger, Gary S. *The Couple's Guide to Fertility*. New York: Doubleday, 1994.

Boston Women's Health Book Collective. *The New Our Bodies, Ourselves*. New York: Simon & Schuster, 1984.

Boyden, T., Pamenter, R., Going, S., et al. Resistance exercise training is associated with decreases in serum low density lipoprotein cholesterol levels in premenopausal women. *Archives of Internal Medicine* 153/1 (1993): 97–100.

Bremer, D. E., et al. Postmenopausal estrogen replacement therapy and the risk of Alzheimer's disease. *American Journal of Epidemiology* 140/3 (1994): 262–67.

Brody, Jane. *Jane Brody's Nutrition Book*. New York: Bantam Books, 1981.

Burger, C., Koomen, L., Peters, N., et al. Postmenopausal hormone replacement therapy and cancer of the female genital tract and the breast. *European Menopause Journal* 1997. On-line *http://www.medscape.com*.

Byyny, Richard, and Speroff, Leon. *A Clinical Guide for the Care of Older Women*. Baltimore: Williams & Wilkins, 1990.

Cabot, Sandra. *Smart Medicine for Menopause*. New York: Avery Publishing Group, 1995.

Carlson, K. J., Eisenstat, S., and Ziporyn, T. *The Harvard Guide to Women's Health*. Cambridge, MA: Harvard University Press, 1996.

Cassidy, A., Bingham, S., and Setchell, K. Biological effects of a diet of soy protein rich in isoflavones on the menstrual cycle of premenstrual women. *American Journal of Clinical Nutrition* 60 (1994): 333–40.

Cauley, Jane A., et al. Estrogen replacement therapy and fractures in older women. *Annals of Internal Medicine* 122/1 (January 1, 1995): 9–17.

Cauley, J., Lucas, F., Kuller, L., et al. Bone mineral density and risk of breast cancer in older women: The study of osteoporotic fractures. *Journal of the American Medical Association* 276 (1996): 1404–08.

Cherry, Sheldon. *The Menopause Book: A Guide to Health and Well-Being for Women After 40*. New York: Macmillan, 1994.

Chopra, D. *Perfect Health*. New York: Harmony, 1991.

Chrischilles, E., Butler, D., et al. A model of lifetime osteoporosis impact. *Archives of Internal Medicine* 151 (1991): 2026–32.

Cobb, J. O. *Understanding Menopause*. New York: Plume, 1993.

Colditz, G. A., Hankinson, S. E., Hunter, D. J., Wilett, W. C., Manson, J. E., Stampfer, M. J., Hennekens, C., Rosner, B., and Speizer, F. E. The use of estrogens and progestins and the risk of breast cancer in postmenopausal women. *New England Journal of Medicine* 332 (1995): 1589–93.

Colditz, Graham A., et al. Hormone replacement therapy and risk of breast cancer: Results of epidemiologic studies. *American Journal of Obstetrics and Gynecology* 168/5 (May 1993): 1473–81.

Collinge, W. *The American Holistic Health Association Complete Guide to Alternative Medicine*. New York: Warner, 1996.

Consumer Reports editors. The estrogen question. *Consumer Reports*, September 1991: 587.

Coronary Drug Project Research Group. The Coronary Drug Project: Initial findings leading to modifications of its research protocol. *Journal of the American Medical Association* 214 (1970): 1303–13.

Cummings, S., Nevitt, M., et al. Risk factors for hip fracture in white women. *New England Journal of Medicine* 332 (1995): 767–73.

Dalton, Katharina. *Once a Month: The Original Premenstrual Syndrome Handbook.* Alameda, CA: Hunter House, 1990.

Doress, P., and Laskin Siegel, D. *Ourselves, Growing Older.* New York: Simon & Schuster, 1987.

Doughty, Susan. Nonhormonal management for menopausal women: Phytoestrogens. *American Menopause Foundation* 3/1 (Summer 1997): 1–4.

Dranov, Paula. *Estrogen: Is It Right for You?* New York: Simon & Schuster, 1993.

Dwyer, Johanna T., et al. Tofu and soy drinks contain phytoestrogens. *Journal of the American Dietetic Association* 94/7 (July 1994): 739–44.

Eisenberg, David. *Encounters with Qi: Exploring Chinese Medicine.* New York: Viking, 1986.

Elias, Marilyn. Mind and menopause. *Harvard Health Letter* 19/1 (November 1993): 1–3.

Ettinger, B., Friedman, G., Bush, T., and Quesenberry, C. P. Reduced mortality associated with long-term postmenopausal estrogen therapy. *Obstetrics and Gynecology* 87 (1996): 6–12.

Ettinger, B., Genant, H., and Cann, C. Long-term estrogen replacement therapy prevents bone loss and fractures. *Annals of Internal Medicine* 102 (1985): 319–24.

Ettinger, B., and Grady, D. The waning effect of postmenopausal estrogen on osteoporosis. *New England Journal of Medicine* 329 (1993): 1192–93.

Felson, D., Zhang, Y., Hannan, M., et al. The effect of postmenopausal estrogen therapy on bone density in elderly women. *New England Journal of Medicine* 329 (1993): 1141–46.

Feskanich, D., Willet, W., Stampfer, M., and Colditz, G. Protein consumption and bone fractures in women. *American Journal of Epidemiology* 143/5 (1996): 472–79.

Foster, Steven. *Field Guide to Medicinal Plants*. New York: Houghton Mifflin, 1990.

Gillespie, Clark. *Hormones, Hot Flashes and Mood Swings*. New York: Harper & Row, 1989.

Gittleman, Ann Louise. *Super Nutrition for Menopause*. New York: Pocket Books, 1993.

Glentzer, Molly. Hot flashes already? *Good Housekeeping*, October 1997: 66–68.

Grady, D., Rubin, S., Petitti, D., et al. Hormone therapy to prevent disease and prolong life in postmenopausal women. *Annals of Internal Medicine* 117/12 (1992): 1016.

Greene, J., and Cooke, D. Life stress and symptoms at the climacterium. *British Journal of Psychiatry* 136 (1980): 486–91.

Greenwood, S. *Menopause Naturally*. Volcano, CA: Volcano Press, 1996.

Grodstein, F., Stampfer, Manson, I., et al. Postmenopausal estrogen and progestin use and the risk of cardiovascular disease. *New England Journal of Medicine* 335/7 (1996): 4523–61.

Harvard Women's Health Watch editors. The latest story on soy. *Harvard Women's Health Watch* 4/9 (May 1997): 6.

——. HRT: An option for the future. *Harvard Women's Health Watch* 4/12 (August 1997): 6.

——. Math + menopause = more questions. *Harvard Women's Health Watch* 4/10 (June 1997): 1–2.

Hendren, John. Race to replace estrogen substitutes. *Associated Press*, September 25, 1997.

Henig, Robin Marantz. *How a Woman Ages: Growing Older, What to Expect and What You Can Do About It*. New York: Ballantine, 1985.

Holzman, G., Ravitch, M., Metheny, W., et al. Physicians' judgments about estrogen replacement therapy for menopausal women. *Obstetrics and Gynecology* 63 (1984): 303–11.

Jacobowitz, Ruth S. *150 Most-Asked Questions About Menopause*. New York: William Morrow, 1993.

JAMA. Effects of estrogen or estrogen/progestin regimens on heart disease risk factors in postmenopausal women: The postmenopausal estrogen/progestin interventions trial. *Journal of the American Medical Association* 273/3 (January 18, 1995): 199–209.

Jovanovic-Peterson, Lois. *A Woman Doctor's Guide to Menopause: Essential Facts and Up-to-the-Minute Information for a Woman's Change of Life*. New York: Hyperion, 1993.

Kitzinger, Sheila. *Birth over Thirty*. New York: Penguin Group, 1995.

Kotz, Deborah. Your period: What's normal, what's not. *Good Housekeeping* 225 (September 1, 1997): 60–62.

Kronenberg, F. Hot flashes: Epidemiology and physiology. *Annals of the New York Academy of Science* 592 (1990): 52–86.

Lamb, Yannic Rice. Winds of the change: Perimenopause tells you that menopause is on the way. *Essence* 26/9 (January 1996): 40–43.

Landau, Carol, Cyr, Michele, and Moulton, Anne. *The Complete Book of Menopause: Every Woman's Guide to Good Health*. New York: G. P. Putnam's Sons, 1994.

Lark, Susan. *The Menopause Self-Help Book*. Berkeley, CA: Celestial Arts, 1992.

Liberman, U., Weiss, R., Broll, J., Minne, H., Wuan, H., et al. Effect of oral alendronate on bone mineral density and the incidence of fractures in postmenopausal osteoporosis. *New England Journal of Medicine* 333/22 (1995): 1437–43.

Love, R., Wiebe, D., Newcomb, P., et al. Effects of tamoxifen on cardiovascular risk factors in postmenopausal women. *Annals of Internal Medicine* 115/11 (1991): 860–64.

Love, Susan. *Dr. Susan Love's Breast Book*. Reading, MA: Addison-Wesley, 1990.

——. *Dr. Susan Love's Hormone Book*. New York: Random House, 1997.

Manson, J., Willett, W., Stampfer, M., Colditz, G., et al. Body weight and mortality among women. *New England Journal of Medicine* 333/11 (1995): 677–85.

Matthews, K., Kuller, L. H., Wing, R. R., Mellahn, E. N., and Plantinga, P. Health prior to use of estrogen replacement therapy: Are users healthier than nonusers? *American Journal of Epidemiology* 143 (1996): 971–78.

McDonnell, D., Clevenger, B., Dana, S., et al. The mechanism of action of steroid hormones: A new twist to an old tale. *Journal of Clinical Pharmacology* 33 (1993): 1165–72.

Melton, L., Eddy, D., and Johnston, C. Screening for osteoporosis. *Annals of Internal Medicine* 112/7 (1990): 516–28.

Meno Times. Report from the 7th Annual North American Menopause Society Meeting. *Meno Times*, December 1, 1996: 16–17.

Messina, Mark. The role of soy products in reducing risk of cancer. *Journal of the National Cancer Institute* 83/7 (1991): 541–45.

——. *The Simple Soybean and Your Health*. New York: Avery Publishing Group, 1994.

Messina, M., et al. Soy intake and cancer risk: A review of the in vitro and in vivo data. *Nutrition and Cancer* 21 (1994): 113–31.

Midlife Woman editors. Yoga at midlife. *Midlife Woman* 5 (January 1, 1996): 11.

Murray, Michael T. *Natural Alternatives to Over-the-Counter and Prescription Drugs*. New York: William Morrow, 1994.

Nash, J. Madeleine. Early flash points: Beset by symptoms caused by ebbing hormones, women in midlife turn to herbs and health foods to smooth out the rocky road to menopause. *Time* 149/16 (April 21, 1997).

National Women's Health Network. Taking hormones and women's health: Choices, risks and benefits. National Women's Health Network, 1993.

Notelovitz, Morris, and Tonnessen, Diana. *Estrogen: Yes or No?* New York: St. Martin's Press, 1993.

——. *Menopause and Midlife Health*. New York: St. Martin's Press, 1993.

Ochs, Ridgely. Prelude to change: Understanding the early symptoms of menopause. *Newsday*, March 25, 1996: 17.

Ojeda, Linda. *Menopause Without Medicine.* Claremont, CA: Hunter House, 1989.

Ornish, D. *Dr. Dean Ornish's Program for Reversing Heart Disease.* New York: Random House, 1990.

Perlmutter, Cathy, Hanlon, Toby, and Sangiorgio, Maureen. Triumph over menopause: Results from our exclusive woman to woman survey. *Prevention* 46 (August 1, 1994): 78–90.

Perry, Susan, and O'Hanlan, Katherine. *Natural Menopause: The Complete Guide.* Reading, MA: Addison-Wesley, 1997.

Peterson, Karen S. Treating symptoms before menopause starts. *USA Today,* April 9, 1996: 4D.

Prevention editors. Menopause naturally. *Prevention,* August 1996: 65–70.

Rako, S. *The Hormone of Desire.* New York: Harmony, 1996.

Reid, I., Ames, R., Evans, M., et al. Effect of calcium supplementation on bone loss in postmenopausal women. *New England Journal of Medicine* 328/7 (1993): 460–64.

Rinzler, Carol Ann. *Estrogen and Breast Cancer: A Warning to Women.* New York: Macmillan, 1993.

Robinson, D., Friedman, L., et al. Estrogen replacement therapy and memory in older women. *Journal of the American Geriatric Society* 42/9 (1993): 2637–41.

Rookus, M, and van Leeuwen, F. Oral contraceptives and risk of breast cancer in women aged 20–54 years. *Lancet* 344/8926 (1994): 844–51.

Sachs, Judith. *What Women Should Know About Menopause.* New York: Dell Publishing, 1991.

Sand, Gayle. *Is It Cold in Here, or Is It Me? Facts, Fallacies and Feelings About Menopause.* New York: HarperCollins, 1993.

Schrotenboer-Cox, Kathryn, and Weiss, J. S. *Pregnancy over Thirty-Five.* New York: Ballantine, 1984.

Seachrist, Lia. What risk hormones? Conflicting studies reveal problems in pinning down breast cancer risks. *Science News* 148/6 (August 5, 1995): 94–95.

Seeman, E., Hopper, J., et al. Reduced bone mass in daughters of women with osteoporosis. *New England Journal of Medicine* 20/9 (1989): 554–58.

Sheehy, Gail. *The Silent Passage.* New York: Random House, 1992.

Sherwin, B. B. Estrogenic effects on memory in women. *Annals of the New York Academy of Science* 743 (1994): 213–30.

Shute, Nancy. Menopause is no disease. *U.S. News & World Report* 122 (March 24, 1997): 71.

Spicer, D., Pike, M., and Henderson, B. The question of estrogen replacement therapy in patients with a prior diagnosis of breast cancer. *Oncology* 4/12 (1990): 49–59.

Stampfer, M. J., Colditz, G. A., Willett, W. C., Manson, J. E., Rosner, B., Speizer, F., and Hennekens, C. H. Postmenopausal estrogen therapy and cardiovascular disease: Ten-year follow-up from the Nurses Health Study. *New England Journal of Medicine* 325/11 (September 12, 1991): 756–62.

Stanford, J. L., Weiss, N. S., et al. Combined estrogen and progestin hormone replacement therapy in relation to risk of breast cancer. *Journal of the American Medical Association* 274/2 (July 12, 1995): 137–42.

Steinberg, Karen K., et al. A meta-analysis of the effect of estrogen replacement therapy on the risk of breast cancer. *Journal of the American Medical Association* 265/15 (April 17, 1991): 1985–91.

Sultenfuss, S., and Sultenfuss, T. *A Woman's Guide to Vitamins and Minerals.* Chicago: Contemporary Books, 1995.

Tanouye, E. Estrogen study shifts ground for women and for drug firms. *Wall Street Journal,* June 15, 1995: A5.

Ulrich, C., Georgiou, C., Snow-Harter, C., and Gillis, D. Bone mineral density in mother-daughter pairs: Relations to lifetime exercise, lifetime milk consumption and calcium supplements. *American Journal of Clinical Nutrition* 63/1 (1996): 72–79.

Valins, Linda. *When a Woman's Body Says No to Sex: Understanding and Overcoming Vaginismus.* New York: Viking, 1992.

Wallis, Claudia. The estrogen dilemma. *Time* 145/26 (June 26, 1995).

Walsh, B., Schiff, I., Rosner, B., et al. Effects of postmenopausal estrogen replacement on the concentrations and metabolism of plasma lipoproteins. *New England Journal of Medicine* 325 (1991): 1196–1204.

Weed, Susun. *The Menopausal Years: The Wise Woman Way*. Woodstock, NY: Ash Tree, 1992.

Weiss, Robert, and Subak-Sharpe, Genell. *The Columbia University's Complete Guide to Health and Well-Being After 50*. New York: Times Books, 1988.

Wright, Karen. Menopause, naturally. *Health,* January–February 1996: 75–79.

Writing Group for PEPI. Effects of estrogen or estrogen/progestin regimens on heart disease risk factors in postmenopausal women. *Journal of the American Medical Association* 273 (1995): 199–208.

Zamarra, J., Schneider, R., et al. Usefulness of the transcendental meditation program in the treatment of patients with coronary heart disease. *American Journal of Cardiology* 77/10 (1996): 867–70.

Ziel, H., and Finkle,W. Increased risk of endometrial carcinoma among users of conjugated estrogens. *New England Journal of Medicine* 293 (1970): 1167–70.

Index